LEPROSY
Diagnosis and Management

Publication Number 871

AMERICAN LECTURE SERIES®

A Monograph in

AMERICAN LECTURES IN DERMATOLOGY

Edited by

JOHN M. KNOX, M.D.

Department of Dermatology
Baylor University College of Medicine
Houston, Texas

LEPROSY
Diagnosis and Management
Second Edition

By

HARRY L. ARNOLD, JR., M.D.

Dermatology Department, Straub Clinic
Clinical Professor of Dermatology
University of Hawaii School of Medicine
Honolulu, Hawaii

and

PAUL FASAL, M.D.

Chief, Leprosy Service
U.S. Public Health Service Hospital
Associate Clinical Professor of Dermatology
University of California School of Medicine
San Francisco, California

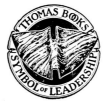

CHARLES C THOMAS • PUBLISHER
Springfield • Illinois • U.S.A.

Published and Distributed Throughout the World by
CHARLES C THOMAS • PUBLISHER
BANNERSTONE HOUSE
301-327 East Lawrence Avenue, Springfield, Illinois, U.S.A.

With THOMAS BOOKS *careful attention is given to all details of
manufacturing and design. It is the Publisher's desire to present books
that are satisfactory as to their physical qualities and artistic possibilities
and appropriate for their particular use.* THOMAS BOOKS *will be true
to those laws of quality that assure a good name and good will.*

First Edition, 1953
Second Edition, 1973

Printed in the United States of America
Q-1

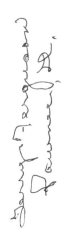

To

Jeanne and Elfriede

PREFACE TO SECOND EDITION

WE ARE at the beginning of a new era in leprosy. We have learned why there are two types of the disease: it is because some patients cannot develop effective cellular immunity against *Mycobacterium leprae*, and hence get progressive leprosy. We have also learned how to tell whether the organisms are alive or dead—by mouse footpad inoculation—and can therefore determine that contagiousness of lepromatous cases diminishes rapidly once treatment is begun.

We have also developed what was only dimly foreseen and hoped for at the time of the first edition: an antibiotic—rifampicin—which rapidly kills *M leprae*.

We have learned that isolation of patients with leprosy is only occasionally, and briefly, advisable; in Hawaii, as a result of this knowledge, it is no longer legally required. Many patients need hospitalization for only a short period for the initiation of treatment, but this often can be done in a general hospital.

No longer, then, does the diagnosis of early leprosy carry with it the threat of complete disruption of a patient's way of life. He can, if his physician is well informed, be managed almost entirely as an outpatient, and can, as a rule, continue to earn a living as he did before.

It is within this almost entirely new framework that we have joined forces to update and expand both the text and illustrations of the first edition of this book, changing its name from *Modern Concepts of Leprosy* to just *Leprosy*.

In keeping with the primarily pragmatic purpose of this book, no bibliography has been included in it. Readers wishing to refer to the literature or wishing advice on a special problem may inquire of either of the authors, or they may write to the USPHS Hospital at Carville, Louisiana 70721, or to The Center for Disease Control in Atlanta, Georgia 30333.

Our observations are directed towards physicians who are not primarily students of leprosy, but general practitioners, dermatologists, or other specialists, who may be faced from time to time with the problem of a patient who appears to have leprosy and who eventually does turn out to have it. Sending patients suffering from leprosy to a remote leprosarium is no longer the order of the day. They may now more often than not remain in the hands of their primary care physician, with advice and guidance from a consultant, or at least return to him after a short period of hospitalization.

To help them to assume this new responsibility is our aim.

HARRY L. ARNOLD, JR., M.D.
PAUL FASAL, M.D.

PREFACE TO FIRST EDITION

IT IS hoped that dermatologists and others may find this monograph a happy medium between the brief chapters on leprosy to be found in most general textbooks and the unnecessarily (for them) detailed accounts found in books devoted exclusively to leprosy. It is written for them, and for students in their field, not for leprologists. I am not a leprologist myself, but a student and practitioner of dermatology who has had the opportunity to see a good many cases of leprosy and to follow some of them over a period of years. I hope that what my background lacks in experience with leprosy will be balanced to some extent by what it gains—for the reader—from the dermatologic point of view. Where this work is too brief or too superficial, it should be supplemented by reference to the practical literature or the texts of Cochrane, Chaussinand, Rogers and Muir, and others. It is not intended to supplant any of these.

I wish to acknowledge my indebtedness to the students of leprosy enumerated in the bibliography, from whose writings I have freely borrowed, and in particular to those who have stimulated my interest and added to my knowledge by personal contact: H. W. Wade, Fernando Latapí, José M. M. Fernandez, Vicente Pardo-Castello, Robert G. Cochrane, F. E. Rabello, Jr., Norman R. Sloan, W. Lloyd Aycock, Edwin K. Chung-Hoon, N. E. Wayson, and my associates, E. A. Fennel and Irvin L. Tilden, of the Pathology Department of the Straub Clinic. It is to Dr. Tilden that I am indebted, too, for the photomicrographs and some of the other photographs, as well as for specific suggestions in the preparation of the manuscript, in which Drs. Fennel, Sloan, Aycock, and Wade were also most helpful.

H. L. A., Jr.

CONTENTS

LEPROSY

Diagnosis and Management

Chapter One

INTRODUCTION

L EPROSY is the most ancient, the most feared, and the most puzzling of all the chronic infectious diseases. For fifteen centuries or more, leprosy was generally considered a highly contagious disease; it was one of the first diseases to be so regarded. Yet students of the disease have known for the past century that in most circumstances, it actually behaves as if it were only very slightly contagious; indeed, vigorous arguments were being waged half a century ago as to whether it was contagious at all or merely hereditary. The late Sir Jonathan Hutchinson wrote a book to prove that leprosy was caused solely by eating imperfectly cured fish, and he died under the shadow of this thoroughly discredited conviction. Now, we believe that leprosy is highly communicable for a very few individuals, but hardly contagious at all for the vast majority of people.

Leprosy is beclouded with other misapprehensions. Old textbooks describe it as manifesting itself in two forms, leprosy of skin and leprosy of nerves. Yet ever since Armauer Hansen, leprosy workers have been aware that each of the two forms of the disease always attacks both skin and nerves.

There are few bacterial diseases in which the causative organism is as easy to find as it is in the lepromatous type of leprosy; yet there are few in which it is as difficult to find as it is in the tuberculoid type (except during reactions).

Many physicians are under the impression—and many textbooks state—that loss of pinprick sensitivity is an early sign of leprosy; actually, it is in many cases a relatively late sign, appearing only after other manifestations of the disease, such as anesthesia to heat or cold, or anhidrosis, have been present for several weeks or months.

It is often stated that the finding of acid-fast bacilli in scrapings or smears from the nasal septum is diagnostic of leprosy—

3

which it is not—and one often encounters the implication that their absence from such preparations rules against a diagnosis of leprosy, which is equally untrue.

Finally, there is a widespread impression in many countries that leprosy is an extremely rare disease, so rare that it is of no great importance. It is not rare; it is uncommon in many areas, but not so rare that it can be ignored. There are perhaps ten million persons in the world who are afflicted with it; and though it is true that the great majority of these live outside the United States, there are still in our country an estimated three thousand known, and many more unrecognized, cases.

The availability of effective treatment imposes a new and grave responsibility upon physicians to be sufficiently alert and well informed to make the diagnosis of leprosy, and make it early, before the disease is so far advanced that irreversible damage has been done. It is primarily to this end that this monograph is dedicated.

Chapter Two

ETIOLOGY

THE causative organism of leprosy is *Mycobacterium leprae*, an acid-fast bacillus described by Dr. Gerhard Armauer Hansen in 1874. It has never been possible to prove its relationship to the disease by fulfilling all of Koch's postulates. The several reports of successful cultivation on artificial media have all failed of confirmation. In 1961, Shepard reported the successful inoculation of lepra bacilli into the footpads of mice. His work has since been widely confirmed. More recently, Kirchheimer and Storrs have been able to inoculate the armadillo successfully. In the mouse, the infection remains limited to the footpad unless the animal has been previously subjected to thymectomy and total body irradiation. In the armadillo, generalized, progressive, systemic leprosy has been observed to occur.

The bacillus is found invariably and in enormous numbers in every lepromatous case of leprosy and in small numbers in a great many cases of the tuberculoid variety of the disease. No doubt is entertained of its being the actual cause of leprosy.

The organism appears in smears or sections as a straight or slightly curved acid-fast rod about 3μ to 5μ long and 0.2μ to 0.4μ thick. When many bacilli occur together, they tend to be aggregated into packets (traditionally likened to "bundles of cigars"), and in much larger aggregates, with spheroid contours, known as globi. It is probable that the latter represent masses of bacilli which have been ingested by (and have multiplied within?) histiocytes, in the course of the generalized granulomatous process which characterizes lepromatous leprosy and accounts for a great many of its curious and characteristic clinical features.

In untreated cases, a high percentage of the bacilli stain solidly from end to end. In cases treated with sulfones for a few weeks, a slowly increasing proportion of the bacilli stain only at each end, or in a discontinuous "granular" or "beaded" fashion throughout their length. The number of solid staining bacilli per one hundred bacilli seen is called the morphologic index or MI, and as it approaches zero the infectivity of the material for mouse footpads also drops to very low levels. It is believed that the beaded bacilli are probably dead, or at least too enfeebled to be infective.

Scores of attempts to transmit leprosy to human volunteers, by inoculating them with fresh, presumably infective material, have almost uniformly failed. The only noteworthy exception, an inoculation of lepromatous tissue made by Edward Arning into the skin of a Hawaiian named Keanu, seems to have been successful. Its importance has been questioned because Keanu is known to have had leprous relatives, and therefore might have been infected by the usual routes; nevertheless, the fact that he developed a leproma at the site of inoculation suggests that the experiment was successful.

The simultaneous occurrence of tuberculoid leprosy in two tattoos received in 1943 by two young American marines from southern Michigan (a wholly nonendemic area) on the same day and in the same shop, in Australia, seems to constitute two more examples of infections of humans by inoculation.

Chapter Three

EPIDEMIOLOGY

THE epidemiology of leprosy is a challenging puzzle, full of
curious paradoxes. Historically, as we have said, leprosy has
been regarded on the one hand as readily communicable, and
on the other hand, as purely hereditary. It is not hereditary, of
course. It is infectious, and communicable, though the degree
of contagiousness ranges from virtually nil, in tuberculoid leprosy with no demonstrable bacilli, to moderately high for susceptible persons in lepromatous leprosy, where bacilli abound.
Susceptibility to infection varies considerably, however, and our
concern here is to examine the factors which influence this, and
to what degree.

AGE

Children have long been regarded as much more susceptible
to leprosy than adults. Cochrane's figures for 2,000 cases seen in
a seven-year period at Chingleput, in Madras, indicate that
about a third of new cases occur before age 15. Chung-Hoon
found in Hawaii that about a third of 316 new cases had their
first reported symptoms before the age of 20. However, the percentage distribution of new cases by age is meaningless unless
one knows the age distribution of the population from which
these cases originated.

In these studies, moreover, as in many similar ones, the only
part of the population not already long exposed to leprosy was
the children. If adults from non-endemic areas had been introduced, they might well have shown an equally high attack rate.
The introduction of leprosy into Netherlands New Guinea in
1960, as reported by Leiker, resulted in the highest attack rate
(39 out of 100) in the 15 to 19 year age group, the next highest
(23 out of 100) in the 10 to 14 year age group; the rate was
15 out of 100 in the 5 to 9 year group, and 16 out of 100 in the

20 to 39 year group. So children were really no more susceptible than adults.

Worth, completing studies begun by Lloyd Aycock on the life history of 642 children born at Kalaupapa Settlement on Molokai and living under a variety of conditions of early exposure to leprosy, came to these conclusions:

1. Living continuously with an untreated lepromatous parent results in leprous infection in about 40 percent of their children, with onset of symptoms between 5 and 14 years of age, and an attack rate in boys about twice as high as that in girls.

2. Infection of children does not occur during the prenatal or intrapartum period: removal of infants at birth is effective in preventing infection.

As Lloyd Aycock pointed out, most infectious diseases are more prevalent among children, and the high incidence of leprosy in children may be in large part a result of their having been exposed within their families, or in scuffling or wrestling with schoolmates, before they grew up. Lara noted that no case of leprosy had yet been seen at Culion among some 600 children of nonleprous employees living in close proximity to the leprosarium. Chung-Hoon found that in about a third of new cases, the disease was first recognized after the age of 40.

Certainly children may be susceptible—but adults may be susceptible, too. There are many instances of leprosy in individuals clearly exposed for the first time in adult life. Age is probably not a determinant of susceptibility to infection with leprosy.

SEX

Leprosy researchers the world over have observed that in general, leprosy is twice as common among males as among females. There are certain curious and perhaps significant exceptions to this remarkably uniform preponderance, however. Hopkins and Faget found no such disparity in Negro admissions to the United States Public Health Service Hospital at Carville, of whom, in a studied period, there were 27 women and 25 men. Rodriguez and Lara, in the Philippines, observed that among children the sexes are attacked equally. Cochrane found that among 5,000 persons examined in Madras, the ratio of males to females was 51:32 (per 1,000) among the adults, and only 77:68 (per 1,000) among the children. Chung-Hoon's figures on 145 newly diagnosed cases of leprosy seen in Hawaii during the period 1945–1949 show a male-female ratio of approximately 2:1 among the lepromatous cases, but only 1.1:1 among those of tuberculoid type.

RACE

It is virtually impossible to evaluate racial susceptibility to leprosy because it can hardly be separated from such other factors as diet, opportunity for contagion, individual inheritance of susceptibility, and so forth. Still, racial variations in incidence are so striking that they deserve mention, whatever the basis for them may be. They are even more remarkable when one considers race in relation to type of leprosy; for example, Cochrane has reported that lepromatous eye lesions were three times as common among Anglo-Indians, in Madras, as among Indians, and laryngeal lesions occurred thirty times as often in the former group as in the latter.

Chung-Hoon has summarized the average morbidity rate in Hawaii by races for a ten-year period, in 316 cases. It ranged from 70.2 (per 100,000 per year) for the Hawaiian group, to 1.1 for the Caucasian (a single case). Part-Hawaiians showed a rate of 13.9 (27 cases), Filipinos 13.6 (20 cases), Chinese 4.3 (eight cases) and Japanese 2.6 (six cases).

OPPORTUNITY FOR INFECTION

Opportunity is also a difficult factor to evaluate in such a disease as leprosy. For example, leprosy workers agree that a bacteriologically negative case—that is, one which no acid-fast bacilli are found in skin lesions—can not transmit the disease to others.

The exact risk of contact with an untreated, bacteriologically positive case—an "open" case—is not known, though we know from Doull's survey in Cebu, and other evidence, that it is many times greater than that of contact with a negative one. Conjugal infection, of one spouse by the other, is notoriously rare. Leprosarium workers are infected very rarely. Yet the relatively high incidence of leprosy in exposed children, described by Cochrane, Lara, and many others, contrasts sharply with the lack of leprosy in children removed at birth from leprous parents, as observed in India, Hawaii, and elsewhere.

Cochrane showed, in an analysis of over 300 cases in which known contact had occurred, that the ratio of room contact to mere house contact was 3:1 for "neural" (chiefly tuberculoid?) cases and over 20:1 for lepromatous cases, suggesting that living in the same room with the latter is potentially dangerous. Lampe and Boenjamin in Indonesia came to exactly the same conclusion.

Kluth reported in 1956 that an epidemiologic survey in Texas had disclosed 40 cases among 1,522 contacts exposed to lepromatous leprosy (2.6%) and only one known case among 495 persons exposed to nonlepromatous leprosy (0.2%). Worth's recent study in Hawaii showed that about 10 percent of Hawaiian or part-Hawaiian children exposed to one or more lepromatous parents, in Hawaii, became infected with leprosy, while no child of a parent known to have tuberculoid leprosy was subsequently found to have been infected.

It is odd, on the face of it, that of Chung-Hoon's series of cases already referred to, approximately 60 percent denied any knowledge of contact with the disease. Moiser, in Africa, reported exactly the same observation. Doull and his associates, in Cebu, obtained no history of contact in 62 percent of cases, and Lampe and Boenjamin, in Indonesia, in 31.4 percent.

Some of these denials must be discounted as untruths. Still, in summary, we must admit that this figure of 30 to 60 percent who deny knowledge of contact, coupled with the rarity of conjugal infection, casts doubt on the oft repeated dictum that prolonged and intimate contact with an "open" case of leprosy is the essential condition for infection. For the highly susceptible person, relatively brief contact may suffice. In the United States, such susceptible persons are rare: most persons probably cannot be infected by any means.

Worth's retrospective study in Hong Kong in 1967 indicated that children exposed to leprous parents already under treatment, however recently treatment was started, are not infected as a result of such exposure. Though the statistical reliability of the results was marginal, they fit so well into the observations of reduction of infectivity for mouse footpads that we consider they may be accepted as valid.

GEOGRAPHIC LOCATION

The curious geographic delimitation of leprosy has long puzzled students of the disease. Its world distribution has varied dramatically during historic time. Our earliest records of it are, like most early medical records, from Africa, India, and China. During the eighth century, it spread into Europe, where it remained prevalent for at least five hundred years, increasing considerably, according to many accounts, during the eleventh, twelfth, and thirteenth centuries. It became comparatively prevalent in the British Isles in the seventh to the ninth centuries, and spread into Scandinavia as well. It is likely that it was spreading eastward from India and China into Oceania during this same period.

From the fifteenth century on, its incidence in Europe, including Great Britain, declined with increasing rapidity, and it has remained definitely endemic only in Africa, India, Burma, South China, Korea, Japan, Central and South America, Mexico, the West Indies, the Malayan archipelago, Okinawa, the Philippines, and many of the Pacific islands. Wherever it exists, it tends to be curiously sporadic, the incidences in villages only a few miles apart often varying widely.

In general, the introduction of new cases of leprosy into previously free areas has not resulted, in the past half century, in the production of new endemic foci. This was true, for example, of Scandinavian immigrants into the North Central United States in the mid-nineteenth century. Only a few secondary cases resulted. In contrast, however, is the remarkable epidemic on the phospate island of Nauru, in the south Pacific, in which the arrival of a single open case was followed by widespread infection of the native population. Norman Sloan found leprosy present and spreading in New Guinea in 1952, though it had been introduced there only about thirty years before.

DIET

Wade has pointed out that leprosy is more prevalent in those parts of China and India where rice is the staple grain, than in areas where "hard" cereals prevail, and the high consumption of rice in Japan and Korea may have a bearing on the relatively high incidence of leprosy in those nontropical countries. The fact that sago is the staple starch in New Guinea is of interest in this connection.

However, relative prosperity, better living conditions, and more hygienic surroundings are more likely to prevail in a wheat-eating population than in one dependent on rice. One can draw no conclusions on the basis of such evidence.

INSECT VECTORS

Bedbugs, fleas, houseflies, mosquitoes, and even cockroaches have been suggested as possible vectors of leprosy. There is so far no proof that any of these, or any other insects, spread the disease, except perhaps by providing bites to be scratched, thus facilitating entry of infection through the skin. Still, the possibility of such transmission exists. For example, the bedbug might well account for the remarkably high risk associated with bed contact as compared to mere room contact.

CLIMATE

It has never been possible to evaluate climatic factors in relation to leprosy, because they cannot be separated from others of greater importance. In general, leprosy seems no longer to be readily transmissible in the temperate zones—that is, those geographic zones characterized by the most intemperate weather—with the notable exception of Japan and Korea. A warm, stable climate seems to be relatively conducive to continued endemicity of the disease. It is the thirtieth parallels of latitude, the world around, that in general define the north and south limits of endemic leprosy today.

TUBERCULOSIS

Chaussinand in several publications advanced the view that tuberculosis and leprosy are antagonistic diseases and that as tuberculosis becomes more prevalent, it tends to promote more widespread resistance to leprosy and so suppress the occurrence of the latter. This view has not been proven. Tuberculosis seems to neither diminish, nor enhance, susceptibility to leprosy.

INHERITED SUSCEPTIBILITY

Danielssen and Boeck, in 1845, put forth the view that leprosy was transmitted solely by inheritance; and despite Hansen's demonstration of the causative organism in 1874, this view retained considerable popularity well into the present century. From the standpoint of explaining observed facts, it had great merit; certainly leprosy did, and does, tend to occur with remarkable frequency among blood relatives, far more so than among those related only by marriage. Among the cases in Cebu in which Doull and his associates were able to get a history of contact, family contacts outnumbered nonfamily contacts by about two to one.

Aycock championed the view that inherited susceptibility to infection explains the seeming discrepancy between the view that the disease is wholly infectious and the view that it is wholly inherited. He was, at the time of his death in 1951, investigating this subject further by genealogic studies among families in Hawaii.

SUMMARY

In conclusion, lepromatous leprosy is certainly transmissible to susceptible persons; close contact with cases of this form of the disease may unquestionably lead to infection, and relatively brief contact may do so for a few highly susceptible individuals.

Chapter Four

NATURAL EVOLUTION OF LEPROSY

O NE OF the most curious and significant properties of *Myco-bacterium leprae* is that it tends either to elicit a vigorous and successful defensive reaction in its involuntary hosts, or else to elicit only an ineffective granulomatous type of reaction. The vigor and degree of success of the defensive reaction may vary somewhat, but it is likely to be, in established cases, either definitely present or definitely absent. Herein lies the basis for the division of cases of leprosy into two "polar" types, as Rabello called them, known at the present time as "lepromatous" (without resistance) and "tuberculoid" (with resistance) respectively. A brief review of the history of the nomenclature of leprosy is most enlightening in this connection.

The most conspicuous, chronic, and generally noticeable type of leprosy is the lepromatous one, as will be seen; and it is primarily this form that was recognized by Greek and Roman physicians under the name "elephantiasis"—chosen, according to Avicenna and Aretaeus, because the disease is "frightening and terrible to look upon, like the elephant" (which was at that time in Europe a beast of war—the tank of the ancients). The names "leontiasis" (from the "lion-like" facies?) and "satyriasis" (from the fancied—and purely imaginary—libidinous tendency of the patient?) are also encountered. Celsus and others wrote also of a disease called "leuce" by the Greeks and "baras" by Arabian physicians, characterized by pale spots and loss of sensation. It is not clear whether leuce was known to be a milder form of elephantiasis; but by the nineteenth century, according to Sir Richard Burton, the Arabs referred to leprosy as occurring in two forms, a mild one known as "baras" and a severe or "red" form known as "juzam."

The word "elephantiasis" remained for several centuries as the specific designation for leprosy, at least of the lepromatous type, with only one modification: the addition of the qualifying *Graecorum* to distinguish it from *elephantiasis Arabum,* or filarial lymphedema of Barbados and other places. No interest was aroused in the classification of leprosy, because in general only lepromatous cases were recognized. The word "leprosy" during this period meant either any scaly disease, or, particularly when used in the Greek form, *lepra,* a nummular variety of psoriasis with central clearing.

The word "lepra" was in turn a translation from the Hebrew word *zaraath*, which at its most specific meant merely any scaly disease, and probably included several (among them, perhaps, leprosy) in its widest sense. It is not apparent that the disease we call leprosy is anywhere specifically referred to in the Bible. It is tragic that the words "lepra" and "leprosy" should ever have been attached to the disease we now know by those names, for with the names have gone all the biblical misconceptions of contagiousness and fear that so harass victims of the disease today.

It was in 1847, with the publication of *Om Spedalskhed* by D. C. Danielssen and Carl Boeck, that the debates over the classification of leprosy began. They named the two forms of the disease "nodular" and "anesthetic," and described also a mixture of these. Their primary criterion for classifying individual cases was the anatomic location of the principal lesions—in the skin in the nodular form, in the nerves in the anesthetic form, and in both in the mixed form. This simple but misleading anatomic classification dominated all thinking about the disease for fifty years, and a great deal of it, including most European and American textbooks, for another fifty.

This is curious, because Gerhard Armauer Hansen, in 1895, published (with Carl Looft) in Norwegian, German, and English a courteous (he was Danielssen's son-in-law) refutation of Danielssen's and Boeck's classification, and put forth his own. His classification was based primarily upon the biologic reaction of the patient to his disease, and was identical with our most modern classification except in its terminology. He called the two types of the disease "lepra tuberosa" and "lepra maculo-anesthetica," and as he said, "we delete altogether the name of mixed leprosy," since each of the two forms of the disease involves both the skin and the nerves, in virtually every case.

Unfortunately, nodular leprosy, as Hansen called it (or lepromatous leprosy, as we call it today), involves the skin relatively early and conspicuously, and the nerves relatively slowly and (except in advanced cases) inconspicuously; and so it came to be thought of by some leprosy workers as a "skin" form of the disease. Maculo-anesthetic leprosy (or tuberculoid leprosy, as we now designate it) usually involves the skin much less conspicuously; and so it came to be thought of by many leprosy workers as a "nerve" form of the disease.

In 1931, at the invitational Leonard Wood Memorial Conference on Leprosy, in Manila, these views were given official expression by an agreement to designate the two forms of leprosy as "cutaneous" and "neural" respectively, with a "mixed" form of leprosy as a subvariety of the "cutaneous" form, characterized by moderately severe nerve damage in addition to the skin lesions. These two forms, cutaneous and neural, were defined in accordance with Hansen's views, not Danielssen's; but the *names* were so simple and clear that there was a tendency to lose sight of the fact that the two types were mutually exclusive, and some workers thereafter classified cases on an almost wholly anatomic basis.

At the First International Congress on Leprosy, in Cairo, in 1938, the Latin American dermatologists made a vigorous effort to gain acceptance of their dualistic classification, which was in effect, as Rabello was to state at Havana in 1948, an expression of Hansen's classification. They were only partially successful. The term "cutaneous" was abandoned in favor of "lepromatous," however, and the term "neural"—though it was, unfortunately, retained—was carefully redefined to include specific skin lesions, the scarcity or absence of bacilli, and the concept of tuberculoid histologic structure as a characteristic feature.

This latter concept, though it had originated with Jadassohn in Europe many years earlier, was surprisingly slow of acceptance by clinical leprologists. Only within the past four decades, thanks largely to the writings of Wade and his co-workers, and of Japanese and Latin American leprologists, has the tuberculoid histologic concept achieved any real standing among leprosy workers. Even at Carville, until about 1945, it was looked upon as an occasionally encountered subdivision of "neural" leprosy.

In 1948, at the Fifth International Congress on Leprosy, in Havana, the tuberculoid concept came of age, and it was agreed to rename the "neural" category "tuberculoid." It was further

TABLE I

HISTORY OF NOMENCLATURE OF LEPROSY

GRECO-ROMAN	Elephantiasis Satyriasis Leontiasis		(Leuce?)
ARABIAN	Juzam		Baras
EARLY EUROPEAN		Elephantiasis Graecorum	
DANIELSSEN & BOECK, 1847		Tubercular leprosy Neural leprosy Mixed leprosy	
MEXICAN circa 1880	Lepra leonina		Lepra antonina
HANSEN 1895	Nodular leprosy		Maculoanesthetic leprosy
MANILA CONFER- ENCE, 1931	Cutaneous leprosy (including "mixed" cases)		Neural leprosy
CAIRO CONGRESS 1938	Lepromatous leprosy		Neural leprosy
HAVANA CONGRESS 1948	Lepromatous leprosy	Indeterminate group	Tuberculoid leprosy
MADRID CONGRESS 1953	Lepromatous type	Borderline group Indeterminate group	Tuberculoid type
TOKYO CONGRESS 1958	No change		
RIO DE JANEIRO CONGRESS 1963	No change		
LONDON CONGRESS 1968	No change		

agreed to acknowledge the existence of a *group* of cases (as distinct from an actual *type* of leprosy) to be designated "indeterminate," on the ground that they could not yet be classified as either lepromatous or tuberculoid. For the Latin American leprologists, this latter category possessed definite characteristics, especially clinically; the British workers especially were inclined to broaden the concept to include cases in transition from one major type to the other ("borderline" cases) and cases unclassifiable for other reasons, for example, because of progression of healing. In 1953, at the Sixth International Congress on Leprosy in Madrid, the borderline group was added. The official definitions of the two types and two groups as developed at this Congress, are shown below. Their schematic relationships are indicated in the following chart.

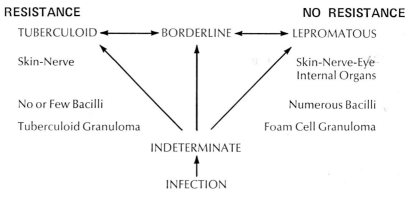

RESISTANCE   NO RESISTANCE

TUBERCULOID ◀━━━━▶ BORDERLINE ◀━━━━▶ LEPROMATOUS

Skin-Nerve   Skin-Nerve-Eye
                                              Internal Organs

No or Few Bacilli   Numerous Bacilli

Tuberculoid Granuloma   Foam Cell Granuloma

INDETERMINATE

INFECTION

OFFICIAL CLASSIFICATION

The following are the official definitions of the two types and two groups of leprosy as developed at the Sixth International Congress of Leprology in Madrid, 1953.

Lepromatous type (L). A malign type, especially stable (as to type, not as to severity), strongly positive on bacteriological examination, presenting more or less infiltrated skin lesions, and negative to lepromin. The peripheral nerve trunks become manifestly involved as the disease progresses, habitually in symmetrical fashion and often with neural sequelae in advanced stages.

Tuberculoid type (T). Usually benign, markedly stable; generally negative on bacteriological examination; presenting in most cases erythematous skin lesions which are elevated marginally or more extensively; positive to lepromin. Sequelae of peripheral nerve trunk involvement may develop in a certain proportion of cases, and this may give rise to serious and disabling deformity. This frequently appears to occur as a result of extension from or through cutaneous nerve branches, rather than of systemic dissemination, and consequently it is often asymmetric and unilateral. Tuberculoid leprosy should be subdivided as follows:

Macular tuberculoid (T_m). These cases present macules with clear-cut and definite margins, the surface generally smooth and dry, invariably with some loss of cutaneous sensibility; almost always negative, or with at most only a few bacilli, on bacteriological examination.

Minor tuberculoid (*micropapuloid*) (T_t). Skin lesions are only slightly to moderately elevated, often only at the margin or even a part of the margin, usually with irregularity of the surface. The condition tends to be relatively superficial, and palpable enlargement of cutaneous nerves associated with the lesion(s) is infrequent.

Major tuberculoid (*plaques, annular lesions, etc.*) (T_T). Skin lesions are often smooth of surface, but more markedly elevated and thickened than in the minor variety, the affected zone usually broader; the more recent lesions may show only partial central recession or no recession; because of the degree of the condition in the deeper levels of the skin, manifest extension in the associated cutaneous nerves is relatively frequent and marked.

Indeterminate group (I). A benign form, relatively unstable, seldom bacteriologically positive, presenting flat skin lesions which may be hypopigmented or erythematous; the lepromin reaction is negative or positive. Neuritic manifestations, more or less extensive, may develop in some cases which have persisted as of this group for long periods. The indeterminate group consists essentially of the "simple macular" cases. These cases may evolve toward the lepromatous type or the tuberculoid type, or may remain unchanged indefinitely.

Borderline (dimorphous) group (B). A malign form, very unstable, almost always strongly positive on bacteriological examination, with the lepromin reaction generally negative. This group may arise from the tuberculoid type as a result of repeated reactions, and sometimes evolves to the lepromatous type. The nasal mucosa is generally bacteriologically negative. The skin lesions are usually seen as plaques, bands, nodules, and so forth, with a regional distribution similar to that of lepromatous leprosy, except for conspicuous asymmetry. The earlobes are likely to present the appearance of lepromatous infiltration. The lesions frequently have a soft or succulent appearance and their periphery slopes away from the center and does not present the clearcut, well-defined margins seen in the tuberculoid type; the lesions are therefore liable to be mistaken for lepromas. The surface of the lesions is generally smooth, with a shiny appearance and a violaceous hue, sometimes (in light skins) with a brownish (sepia) background.

Plate 1A. Lepromatous leprosy: macular exanthematic eruption, trunk.

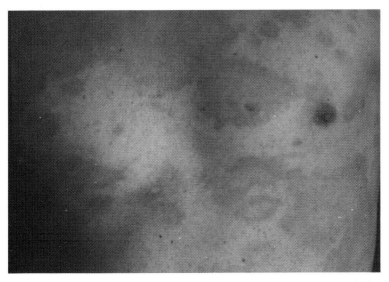

Plate 1B. Lepromatous leprosy: erythematous plaques, simulating seborrheic dermatitis.

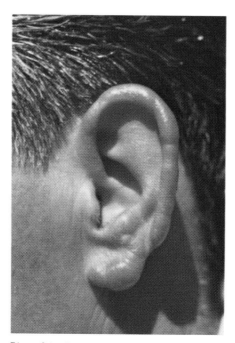

Plate 2A. Lepromatous leprosy: nodules and infiltration, both ears.

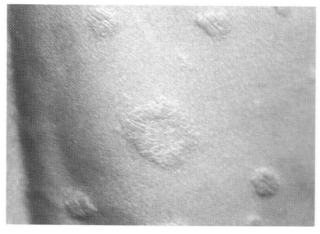

Plate 2B. Lepromatous leprosy, toward borderline: plaques with steep inner border and gently sloping periphery.

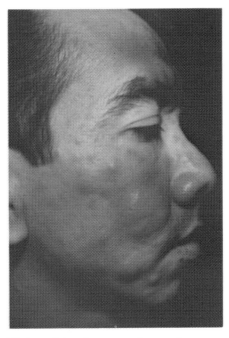

Plate 3A. Lepromatous leprosy: nodules, various sizes, face, treated for years as acne conglobata.

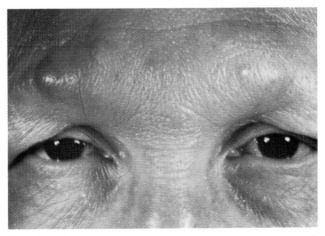

Plate 3B. Lepromatous leprosy: loss of eyebrows and nodules of forehead.

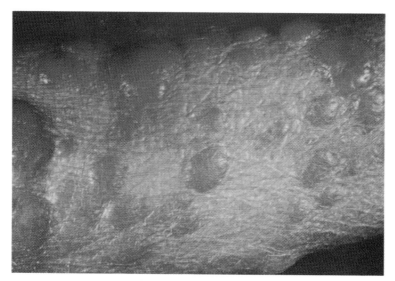

Plate 4A. Lepromatous leprosy: tumor-like masses, forearm.

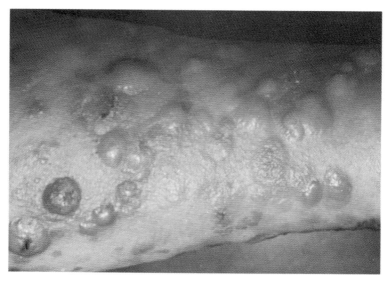

Plate 4B. Reticulum cell lymphoma: tumor-like masses, forearm.

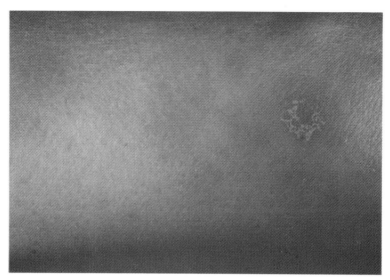

Plate 5A. Erythema nodosum leprosum: red subcutaneous nodules next to old lesions, pigmented, with fine scales.

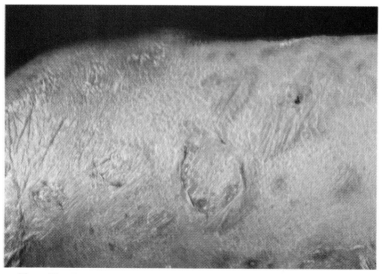

Plate 5B. Lepromatous leprosy: bullous multiforme-like reaction.

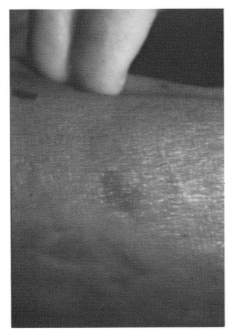

Plate 6A. Diffuse lepromatosis: early erythema necroticans.

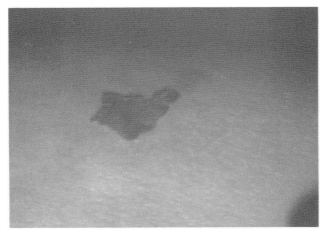

Plate 6B. Diffuse lepromatosis: black eschar in erythema necroticans. See Figures 11 and 12.

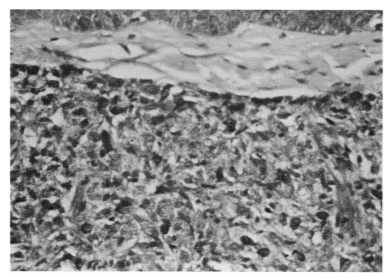

Plate 7A. Lepromatous leprosy, acid-fast stain. Note free "grenz" zone between epidermis and granuloma.

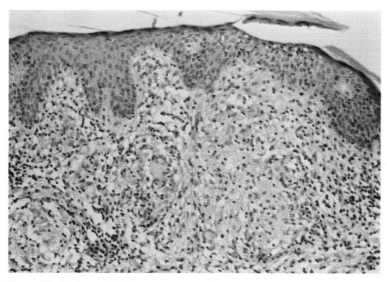

Plate 7B. Tuberculoid leprosy: granuloma in upper corium, touching the epidermis.

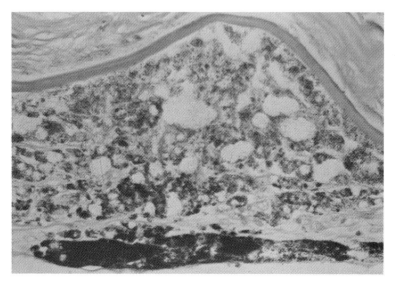

Plate 8A. Lepromatous leprosy, eye, invasion of ciliary body by innumerable bacilli.

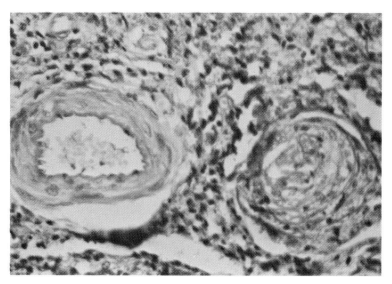

Plate 8B. Lepromatous leprosy, acid-fast stain: selective nerve involvement.

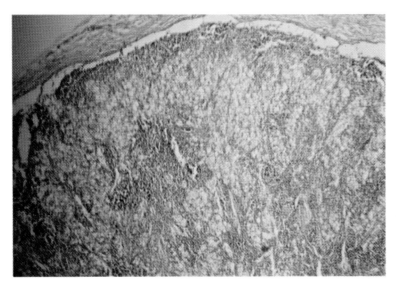

Plate 9A. Lepromatous leprosy, lymph node: replacement of normal tissue by foam cells.

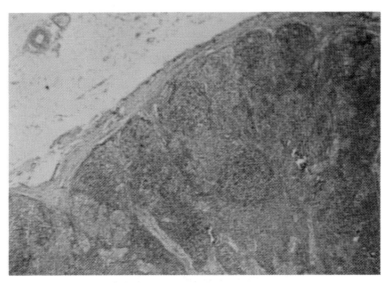

Plate 9B. Lepromatous leprosy: lymph node, aicd-fast stain. More abundant bacilli.

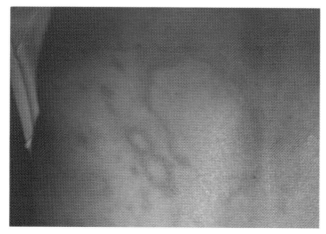

Plate 10A. Borderline leprosy: gyrate lesions with elevated borders.

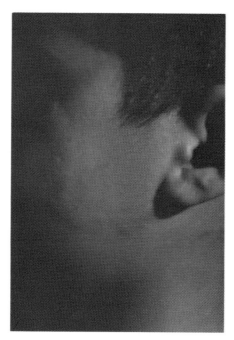

Plate 10B. Borderline leprosy: sharp border inside, sloping outside.

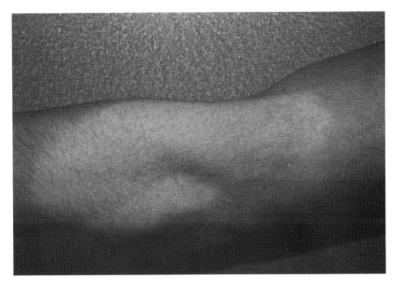

Plate 11A. Tuberculois leprosy: large hypopigmented lesion, elbow.

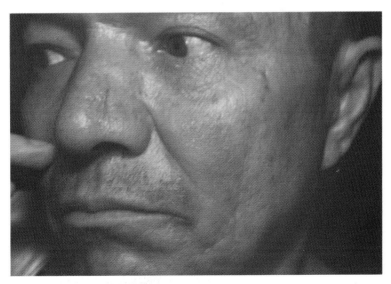

Plate 11B. Tuberculoid leprosy (major): infiltrated red plaque, left side of face.

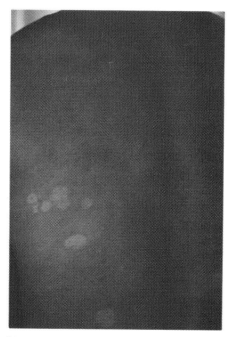

Plate 12A. Tuberculoid leprosy and sharply demarcated tinea versicolor of lower back. Irregular plaque, elevated border, shoulder.

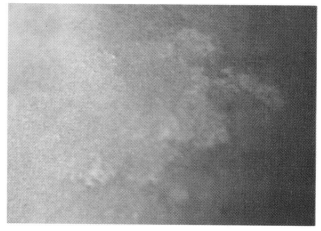

Plate 12B. Close-up of A.

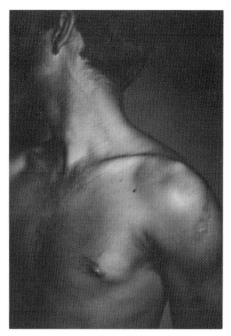

Plate 13A. Tuberculoid leprosy (plaque, left chest) with enlarged great auricular nerve.

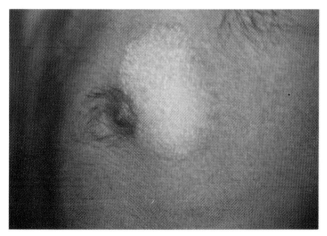

Plate 13B. Tuberculoid leprosy, close-up of A, hypopigmented center, elevated border.

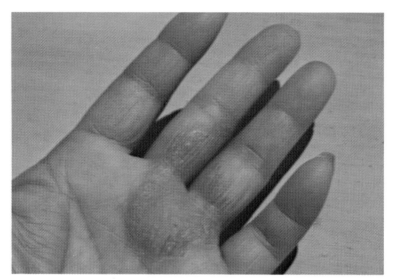

Plate 14A. Tuberculoid leprosy simulating tinea: vesicular border.

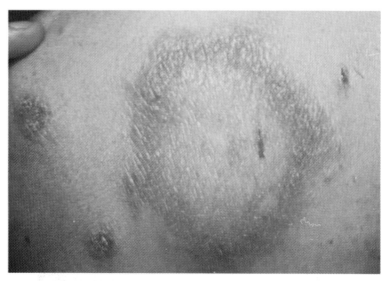

Plate 14B. Tuberculoid leprosy: reddish-brown, elevated, annular plaque.

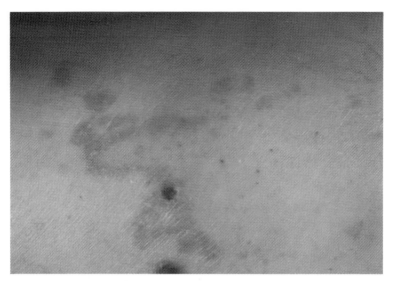

Plate 15A. Tuberculoid leprosy: serpiginous lesion, simulating late syphilis.

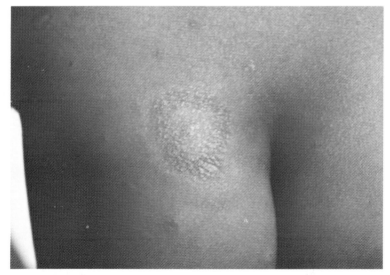

Plate 15B. Borderline-tuberculoid leprosy, "cockade" pattern.

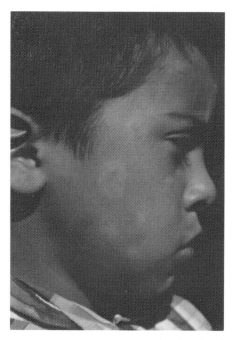

Plate 16A. Follicular mucinosis simulating tuberculoid leprosy. Slight anesthesia present. Biopsy was diagnostic.

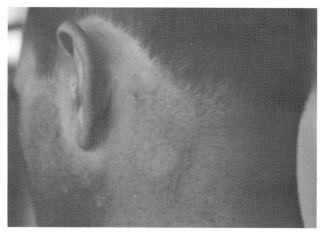

Plate 16B. Elastosis perforans simulating tuberculoid leprosy.

Chapter Five

THE DIAGNOSIS OF LEPROSY

SUSPICION

EVEN advanced cases of leprosy may sometimes prove difficult to recognize. In early cases, where nerve involvement is not obvious, the diagnosis may not even be considered. There is no substitute for a high index of suspicion. A survey of the more important skin lesions which should arouse suspicion may be helpful.

Norman Sloan, in a review of 743 cases in which presenting symptoms were recorded, found that nearly half of these were described by the patients as spots or blotches, usually pale, but occasionally hyperpigmented or reddened. The appearance may be essentially the same as that of *tinea versicolor* (Plate 12A) though the dusty scaliness of the latter is seldom noted, and there is little tendency to the "continent-with-surrounding-islands" pattern of distribution of the fungus infection. *Tinea* may be closely simulated (Plate 14A), even to the central clearing (Figs. 1 and 2) but scaling and itching seldom occur. *Vitiligo* is imitated only superficially (Plates 11, 12 and 13); complete depigmentation never occurs in leprosy (except in scars). Leprous lesions are merely hypopigmented. *Seborrheic dermatitis* may be imitated (Plate 1B), but rarely in just the seborrheic sites of involvement. *Pityriasis rosea* may be simulated so closely as to confuse even the expert eye; and long persistence, occasional associated anesthesia, or thickening of nerves may be the only clinical clues. The pale facial macules of *pityriasis alba* (also known as "pityriasis simplex," "impetigo sicca," "erythema streptogenes," or "achromia parasitica"), are distinguishable from macules of leprosy only with difficulty, by their fine scaliness and by a lack of evidence of leprosy. Anesthesia is not found, but it is notoriously slow to develop on the face in leprosy. We have never seen

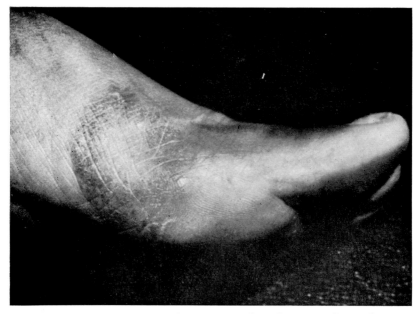

FIGURE 1. Minor tuberculoid leprosy: annular plaque, with tactile anesthesia. Palpable nerve trunk entering it from left top.

one of these cases eventuate in leprosy; all appear either to respond to treatment or to recover spontaneously.

The hypopigmented macules of *follicular mucinosis* (alopecia mucinosa), especially if the characteristic "nutmeg-grater" configuration is inconspicuous or absent, may closely simulate, or be simulated by, leprosy, (Plate 16A). The differentiation is especially difficult because hypesthesia or actual anesthesia to cold, and even anesthesia to touch, may be found in lesions of follicular mucinosis.

Psoriasis may mimic leprosy. The fully developed psoriatic lesion, with its silvery, lamellated scale, rarely occurs as a manifestation of leprosy, however, especially in the typical psoriatic sites. It is only atypical psoriasis that should arouse suspicion.

Lupus erythematosus may be imitated by leprosy, though here again it is an imperfect imitation. Typical, fully developed lesions of *discoid lupus erythematosus* need not occasion any special concern.

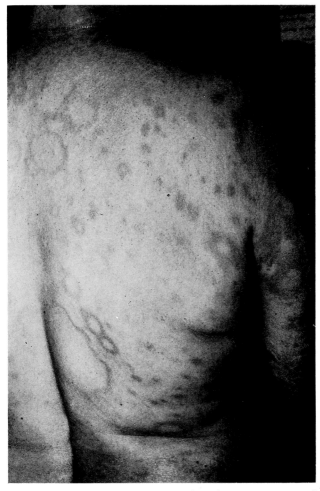

FIGURE 2. Borderline leprosy, generalized though asymmetric, with annular plaques. No anesthesia in lesions. Bacilli present. BL subgroup: tending toward lepromatous.

Almost one-fourth of Sloan's series of cases began with "lumps," nodules, or swellings. A common erroneous diagnosis in such cases is *urticaria,* or, less often, *erythema nodosum* or *erythema multiforme.* It should be noted, however, that both erythema nodosum (Plate 5A) and genuine erythema multiforme (Plate 5B) of almost any type, including the bullous, may actually be caused by leprosy; it may occur as part of the febrile allergic flare-up known as the lepra reaction (see page 000).

Early lesions of lepromatous leprosy may also, however, resemble urticarial wheals so closely as to deceive an experienced physician into treating a patient for hives. It is therefore important to beware of cases of *urticaria* in which the "wheals" are persistent instead of transitory and the patient complains of skin lesions but not of itching.

Another nodular disorder sometimes misdiagnosed in the presence of leprosy is *neurofibromatosis*; lepromas are not always red and may closely imitate neurofibromas. Lepromas do not "buttonhole"—that is, drop easily into the underlying fatty panniculus on finger-pressure, as neurofibromas characteristically do.

Granuloma annulare may be imitated by leprous lesions; so may *xanthomatosis, mycosis fungoides,* other *lymphomas* (Plate 4), cutaneous *leukemia* (especially *monocytic*), late non-ulcerative *syphilis* (Plate 15A), and *sarcoidosis.*

The last deserves special mention, because the histologic changes in *Boeck's sarcoid* and in tuberculoid leprosy may be so similar that a histologic error in diagnosis may confirm a clinical error. The most reliable way to distinguish tuberculoid leprosy from *sarcoidosis* is by testing the skin lesion for evidence of deficient innervation, which will almost invariably be present in this form of leprosy in the skin (except rarely in some facial lesions), and will not be present in any case of sarcoidosis. Hyperglobulinemia is not usually present in tuberculoid leprosy. Histologically, in leprosy, nerve involvement is distinctive.

Erysipelas—but without fever—is so exactly imitated by many a case of tuberculoid leprosy in reaction, or in borderline leprosy, that it is not rare for leprous patients to be hospitalized with that diagnosis. In the presulfonamide era the error usually became apparent by the second or third day, when the physician or an alert intern noticed the absence of fever and leukocytosis; but nowadays, when the patient with erysipelas is expected to be afebrile after the first few hours, the error may be expected to go unnoticed a little longer. Differentiation is made additionally difficult by the fact that anesthesia may develop relatively late

67452

in facial lesions, sometimes only after they have been present for several weeks. Associated thickening of nerve trunks, or biopsy, may help to avoid such errors.

MISCELLANEOUS SKIN AND MUCOSAL CHANGES

Loss of the lateral portions of the eyebrows, though not an early sign, is an important manifestation of lepromatous infiltration (Plate 3B). It is usually symmetrical, and differs in no essential respect from Fournier's "signe d'omnibus" of *syphilis.* In pure diffuse "spotted" leprosy of Lucio (see Chapter Six) this is the only obvious external evidence of the disease (prior to the appearance of the "spots"). In more advanced stages, the eyelashes and body hair are lost as well.

Eye lesions, though they occur only in advanced lepromatous cases, should arouse suspicion. *Episcleritis, pannus* formation, *keratitis,* and *iridocyclitis* (Plate 8A) may occur in lepromatous leprosy. In the tuberculoid type, and in children, one should be alert to such inconspicuous features as widening of the palpebral fissure by slight ptosis of the lower lid, usually on only one side, or less often, its narrowing by ptosis of the upper lid. Later, lagophthalmos (inability to close the lids) is characteristic (Fig. 3).

Hoarseness from leprous involvement of the larynx may be a useful clue to diagnosis. It is a late sign, however.

Lupus vulgaris and *tuberculosis verrucosa cutis* may be imitated by leprosy, though the reverse is more often true. *Erythema induratum,* various tuberculids, or *scrofuloderma* may also be simulated. This mimicry is particularly important because even an experienced pathologist may occasionally mistake the tuberculoid histologic structure for the tuberculous one.

Drug eruptions, dermatitis factitia, foreign-body granuloma, ichthyosis, leishmaniasis, lichen planus (Fig. 4), *neurotic excoriations,* and *pinta* are a few additional conditions which may be mistaken for leprosy—or vice versa. Remember that leprosy lesions rarely itch, ulcerate, lichenify, or scale!

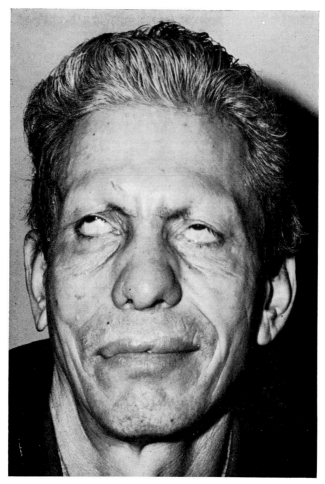

FIGURE 3. Lepromatous leprosy "treated" for seventeen years as syringomyelia. Note loss of eyebrows, lagophthalmos, and sagging right oral commisure.

NEUROLOGIC CHANGES

Nearly a fifth of Sloan's series reported neurologic changes as the initial manifestation of their disease, and foremost among such changes is, of course, "numbness" or anesthesia of the skin. Circumscribed tactile anesthesia of the skin is due to leprosy more often than not, though the diagnosis may have to depend in such cases on (a) demonstration of characteristic histologic

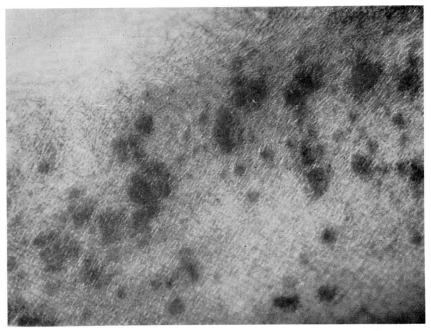

FIGURE 4. Lepromatous leprosy: generalized eruption of flat, dark-red, papular lesions simulating lichen planus.

changes in biopsy specimens, sometimes only in the subcutaneous tissues; (b) demonstration of leprous involvement of thickened nerve trunks, either nearby or elsewhere; or (c) eventual progression of the numb area into a full-blown tuberculoid plaque over a period of weeks or months.

A common nonleprous cause of circumscribed numbness, which should be kept in mind, is so-called *meralgia paresthetica,* or Bernhardt's disease—a numb area on the outside of the thigh presumed to be due to pinching of the lateral femoral cutaneous nerve where it traverses the fascia lata or the inguinal ligament. This is often associated with intermittent neuralgia in the same nerve, either spontaneous, or elicited by weight-bearing on the affected leg. In at least three instances, to our knowledge, this syndrome has made leprologists fear they had acquired leprosy.

Other *peripheral neuritides* (diabetic or alcoholic, for example) may cause confusion, but bear in mind that they rarely cause anesthesia, and that leprous neuritis only very rarely, and in its most advanced degrees, causes loss of tendon reflexes. Diabetic neuropathy may duplicate the neurotrophic bone changes, especially in the feet, which we associate with leprosy. Thickening of nerve trunks, however, especially if nodular, is rarely on any other basis than leprosy. Beware of dismissing glove or stocking anesthesia as hysterical; this pattern is very common in moderately advanced leprosy, especially of the lepromatous type.

Malum perforans is a characteristic complication of leprous neuritis: a painless, indolent plantar ulcer with hyperkeratosis of the surrounding skin is due to leprosy more often than to *diabetes, tabes dorsalis,* or, of course, *syringomyelia.* Such an ulcer is not a leprous lesion, any more than it is a syphilitic one in tabes: it is purely trophic, and neither bacteriologic nor histologic evidence of the causative disease will be found in it.

The appearance of *syphilitic dactylitis* may be suggested by vasomotor paralysis in the skin of the hands. Such lesions are usually symmetric, and characterized by a dusky cyanotic hue, puffiness of the fingers, and warmth.

Syringomyelia, though rare, is usually characterized (like leprosy) by sensory dissociation—that is, anesthesia to pain or cold, or both, in areas where tactile sensation is preserved. The differential diagnosis should not be unduly difficult; but if it is, it may be clarified by tests designed to determine whether nerve damage has occurred in the skin (as it does in leprosy) or only centrally (as in syringomyelia). The histamine test of Rodriguez; or the intradermal injection of pilocarpine, acetylcholine, or methacholine, to elicit sweating; or of nicotine salts, to elicit a pilomotor response, will serve this purpose.

Facial paralysis of the sort described as *Bell's palsy* must be rare in leprosy, as Cochrane observed, especially without other evidence of the disease. As Monrad-Krohn has pointed out in his authoritative monograph on the neurologic changes of leprosy, facial weakness and paralysis in leprosy are almost always partial, and often bilateral but asymmetric.

Traumatic neuritis, as from injury to the ulnar nerve, can usually be differentiated on the basis of lack of sensory dissociation, lack of other evidence of leprosy (including thickening of the nerve), and the history.

PROOF

The diagnosis of leprosy is a serious matter, and strong suspicion of its correctness is neither medically nor socially adequate. The consequences of the diagnosis can be so serious and far-reaching that it is vital to secure absolute proof that it is correct.

The minimal diagnostic criteria for leprosy are either (a) acid-fast bacilli morphologically consistent with *M leprae* and found in such a place* that they may reasonably be assumed to be that organism; or (b) histologic evidence of nerve involvement.

In many cases, *only one of these criteria can be satisfied—not both.*

This latter point is frequently ignored, with the result that cases of leprosy are missed. As indicated in Tables II and III, lepromatous and tuberculoid leprosy differ sharply from one another in a great many respects, and here is one of the most important. In untreated *lepromatous* leprosy, bacilli will always be found in the skin lesions (Plate 7) but clinically demonstrable nerve damage is likely to be lacking altogether in very early cases. In *tuberculoid* leprosy, nerve damage of some slight degree will almost always be demonstrable, but bacilli are likely to be absent, except during reactions.

So when minimal diagnostic criteria are considered, it is vital to decide in advance whether they are being applied to a suspected lepromatous case, or to a suspected tuberculoid one. *Lepromatous leprosy cannot be excluded* on the ground that *cutaneous sensation is not disturbed, and tuberculoid leprosy cannot be excluded* on the ground that *bacilli are not found.*

Finally, a diagnostic histologic picture—with either acid-fast bacilli, or nerve involvement, or both—should be included as part of the minimal requirements for diagnosis.

---

* That is, not in open ulcers, smegma, or nasal scrapings, or on the skin surface.

TABLE II

LEPROMATOUS LEPROSY VS. TUBERCULOID LEPROSY

Clinical Features	Lepromatous	Tuberculoid
Sites of election	Skin (and nerves)	Nerves (and skin)
Visceral lesions	Many subclinical	(lymph nodes?)
Mucosal lesions	Often and early	Nose only
Eye lesions	Often, late	Rarely
Pale macules	Sometimes	Frequently
Annular plaques	Sometimes	Frequently
Erythema multiforme	In reactions	Not seen
Erythema nodosum	In reactions	Not seen
Fever	In reactions	Not seen
Eyebrow alopecia	Common	Not seen
Gynecomastia	May occur, late	Not seen
Symmetry of lesions	Common	Often lacking
Nerve enlargement	Slow, symmetric	Rapid, asymmetric
Nerve damage	Slow	Rapid
Anesthesia	Glove and stocking	In macules or plaques; circumscribed

Histologic Features		
General pattern	Xanthoma-like	Sarcoid-like
Lymphocytes	Few	Numerous
Giant cells	Occasional; foreign body or Touton	Often; Langhans type
Lipoid	Abundant	Minimal
Necrosis	Rare	Rare except in nerves
Nerve changes	Fibrosis; structure well preserved	Normal architecture obliterated early
Visceral amyloidosis	Common (late)	Not seen

Bacterioscopy		
Acid-fast bacilli	Always abundant	Rare except in reactions

Immunology		
Cellular immunity	Very low	High
Humoral immunity	High	Low
Lepromin reaction	Mitsuda negative	Mitsuda positive
False positive serology	40-60 per cent	None

Course		
Untreated	Progression	Spontaneous recovery often

SEARCH FOR BACILLI

The simplest method of looking for bacilli in skin lesions is Wade's "scraped incision" method, sometimes called a "snip." The edge of an earlobe, or a fold of skin at the margin of a skin lesion, or on any acral part, is pinched firmly and incised with a new No. 15 Bard-Parker blade to a depth of about 2 mm and for a length of 5 or 6 mm (Fig. 5). The side of the cut thus made is scraped repeatedly with the edge of the blade (Fig. 6) until a good-sized drop of cloudy tissue juice and pulp is obtained. This is then spread on a new microscope slide over an area about 15 mm in diameter, allowed to dry, and stained by the Fite Faraco method.

A rough approximation to a quantitative count, which is called the bacteriological index (BI) may be made as follows:

    1 to 10 bacilli per 100 oil-immersion fields, BI=1
    1 to 10 bacilli per 10 oil-immersion fields, BI=2
    1 to 10 bacilli per oil-immersion field, BI=3

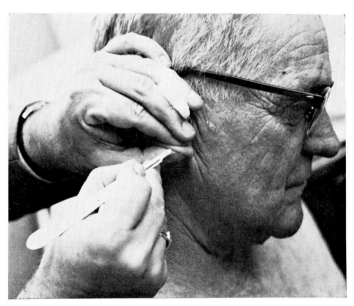

FIGURE 5. Obtaining tissue juice from an earlobe by the scraped incision technique: making the incision.

10 to 100 bacilli per oil-immersion field, BI=4
100 to 1000 bacilli per oil-immersion field, BI=5
over 1000 bacilli per oil-immersion field, BI=6

A further determination known as the morphologic index, or MI, is made by counting the number of solid-staining bacilli per 100 organisms seen; it is believed that such organisms are the only viable, potentially infective ones. This is difficult: it requires an excellent microscope and light source, and a specially trained technician, and even then the readings are not closely comparable with readings in other laboratories, only with those in the same laboratory.

The practical value of the "snip" for the diagnosis of leprosy is limited, as only a positive finding is significant. If the scraping is negative, the patient may have (a) tuberculoid leprosy; (b) active lepromatous leprosy with a zone of normal connective tissue between epidermis and granuloma so wide (Fig. 28) that

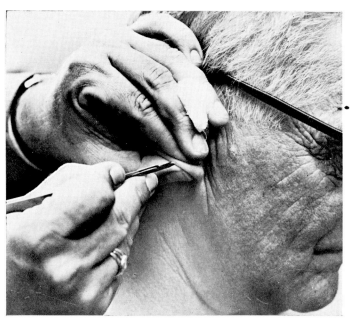

FIGURE 6. Obtaining tissue juice by scraped incision: scraping the side of the cut. Note that the scalpel has been turned at a right angle.

the scalpel did not reach the bacillus- containing layer; (c) lepromatous leprosy in a late stage when no bacilli are present in the skin lesions, but characteristic tissue changes do exist; or (d) not leprosy, but some other disease (perhaps as serious as leprosy). In all four situations, histopathological examination of a biopsy specimen will give the answer, which a "scraped incision" does not do.

We feel it is essential to perform a biopsy in all suspected cases of leprosy. The method of obtaining the skin specimen is of no importance, as long as we obtain a sufficiently deep sampling of all the layers of the skin. Punch biopsies are generally preferable to scalpel excisions on account of the greater simplicity of the procedure. Cutaneous punches 4 to 6 mm in diameter are suitable.

Of greatest importance is the selection of the site for the biopsy. It should always be obtained from an area with the greatest activity. The lesion should be a relatively fresh or active one, and the specimen should not contain affected and normal skin, but only affected skin. If a punch biopsy specimen contains half affected and half normal skin, the sections may easily only show normal skin. In a lesion which has been enlarging, the punch should be placed close to the border of the lesion, but still completely within it.

There are two situations when we do have to perform a biopsy of normal-appearing skin. In lepromatous as well as in tuberculoid leprosy, without any apparent skin lesions, a specimen obtained from normal-appearing skin in a hypesthetic area may show definite nerve involvement and sometimes even granulomatous changes. In diffuse lepromatosis, the only clinical manifestation may be loss of hair, especially eyebrows and eyelashes. The only subjective complaint may be numbness of the extremities. In such a case we perform a biopsy of normal-appearing skin, and we usually find, in such a specimen, numerous bacilli.

For anesthesia, we usually use local infiltration with procaine or xylocaine® solution (1%) with as small a needle as possible (30 gauge). If pain sensation is lost, the biopsy of course can be performed without any local anesthetic. The punch must be sharp; it should be held perpendicular to the skin and rotated, with slight pressure. One can feel when the instrument penetrates the corium and "falls" into the subcutis. Often it is possible to lift out the specimen with a forceps without any difficulty, as the fatty tissue of the subcutis is usually very loose. However, a pair of small, sharp scissors should be available to separate the skin specimen from the deeper fatty layers. It is important not to crush the specimen: hold it gently with a fine forceps or hook. Transfer it immediately to a labeled container containing a 10% formalin solution.

If a 4-mm punch is used, it is seldom necessary to suture the wound, except on the face. When using a 6-mm punch, it is usually advisable to use one or two sutures for closure, to control bleeding, speed healing, and minimize scarring.

Leprosy is a great imitator, not only clinically, but also histopathologically. If one suspects leprosy in a biopsy specimen, all available facts should be presented to the examiner, and it is advisable as well to select a pathologist or dermatopathologist familiar with leprosy.

A word of warning is in order with regard to the examination of nasal scrapings. The nasal mucous membrane may harbor acid-fast bacilli which are morphologically very similar indeed to *M leprae*. Eskey, in Honolulu, cultivated such organisms repeatedly from nasal scrapings from patients at the Kalihi Receiving Hospital, and we have found them in nonleprous "suspects" on more than one occasion. Conversely, the nasal mucous membrane may show no acid-fast bacilli in as many as two-thirds of early lepromatous cases. For purposes of diagnosis, therefore, nasal scrapings are of little or no value to the expert and may seriously mislead the inexperienced.

SEARCH FOR NERVE DAMAGE

The patient's face and hands should be inspected for asymmetry caused by weakness or atrophy of muscles. The face should be examined *in repose* for such features as a widened palpebral fissue, a drooping upper or lower lid (Fig. 3), or a drooping oral commissure. Efforts to smile or raise the eyebrows are apt to efface, rather than emphasize, these early manifestations of muscular weakness. One or both hands may show tapering of fingertips, flattening of thenar or hypothenar eminences, grooving between the metacarpals, slight flexion contracture of the fifth finger, or in more advanced lesions, external rotation of the thumb and finally the characteristic "simian" or even "claw" hand so often seen in the advanced case (Fig. 7).

Palpation for thickened, nodulated, stiffened, or tender nerve trunks is the next step. The nerves most easily examined are the great auricular nerves, which can be felt in most thin normal persons as they cross the sternocleidomastoid muscles, running from the midpoints of these posteriorly, upward and forward toward the angle of the jaw, parallel to, and an inch or so above and behind, the external jugular vein. Asymmetric thickening is especially significant; if marked, it is virtually diagnostic (Fig. 8). The ulnar nerves are even more readily felt, though it is often difficult to be sure whether they are abnormal or not, especially if they are symmetrically involved. The common peroneal, pos-

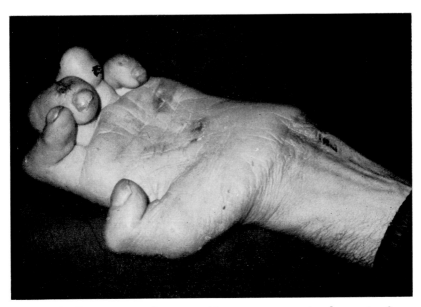

FIGURE 7. Lepromatous leprosy with severe nerve involvement. Same patient as Fig. 3. Note contracture of all digits ("claw" hand) and external rotation of thumb ("simian" hand), with atrophy of thenar and hypothenar eminences.

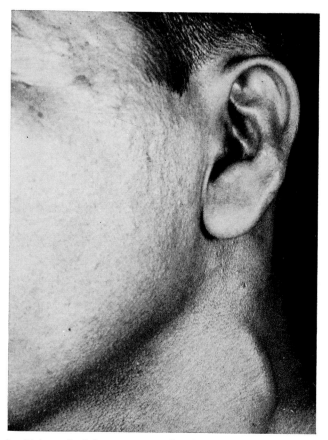

Figure 8. Tuberculoid leprosy: greatly thickened great auricular nerve. Only a small inconspicuous skin lesion was present, and there was no anesthesia.

terior tibial, sural, radial, median, and supraorbital nerves are not infrequently involved, either in their main portions or in their superficial cutaneous branches. Nerves in the vicinity of tuberculoid skin lesions are especially apt to be thickened, often conspicuously so.

Trophic changes in bone may also provide evidence of nerve damage; concentric absorption of the shafts of phalanges, metatarsals, or (rarely) metacarpals, or in more advanced cases, actual loss of continuity of the shafts, results in shortening (*not* dropping off) of digits (see Fig. 9).

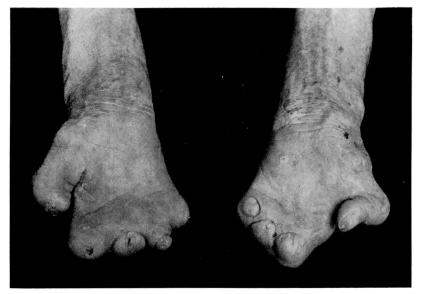

FIGURE 9. Lepromatous leprosy with severe symmetrical nerve damage and trophic absorption of the phalanges. Note persistence of fingernails on remaining stumps.

Lack of sweating characterizes even the earliest lesions of leprosy, and may be detected, especially on the hands, before anesthesia is noted. It was said of Father Damien's original skin lesions that "the perspiration did not appear upon them as elsewhere."

Anesthesia of the skin, either of glove and stocking type in a lepromatous case, or of the skin lesions (or other areas) in a tuberculoid one, should be looked for. Tactile anesthesia, though it is seldom the earliest form to appear, is most easily demonstrated, often by merely touching the skin as lightly as possible with the ball of the examiner's middle finger. Should this fail to demonstrate anesthesia, a small camel's-hair brush, or, as recommended by Ryrie, a wisp of cotton, should be tried, always comparing sensation within the lesion with sensation outside it. Bear in mind that, while loss of tactile sensation in a skin lesion is almost diagnostic of leprosy, *preservation* of tactile sensation is of *no* significance.

Pinprick anesthesia or hypesthesia, though it usually appears after the sense of touch has gone, may be present quite early, and is worth looking for. *Preservation* of the sense of pain or of sharpness, like that of touch, is of no significance.

Thermal anesthesia—inability to identify either hot or cold stimuli, or both—is likely to be more widespread, and more consisently present, than either tactile anesthesia or analgesia. *It should always be looked for in suspicious lesions when tactile sensation appears to be preserved.* It can be tested for by using test tubes containing melting ice, and water at about 100°F, respectively. Too hot water is to be avoided because contact with it may be identifiable as painful. The patient should be asked to distinguish the warm stimuli from the cold ones, and his ability to do this inside the lesions, and in the normal surrounding skin, should be compared. An occasional correct response within the lesion, like an occasional wrong one outside it, is not reassuring if there is decidely diminished accuracy in the former area as compared with the latter.

Frequently it happens that only one or two types of anesthesia will be found in a given area; such sensory dissociation is common in leprosy. Occasionally no anesthesia will be found, or perhaps the sensory changes will suggest syringomyelia. In either of these events, either a histamine test or a methacholine sweating test may be used to carry the examination further.

The histamine test, originally described in 1931 by Rodriguez and Plantilla, is a sensitive objective test for intracutaneous nerve damage. A small drop of 1:1000 solution of histamine diphosphate is placed on the skin inside the area to be tested and another drop outside. A superficial pinprick is then made through each drop. A wheal will then form at each puncture site; but the red flare which forms about the wheal in the normal skin will be lacking about the wheal in the involved area, if intracutaneous nerves have been destroyed. In syringomyelia, as in normal persons, both wheals will be surrounded by a flare. Should dermatographia be present, as it sometimes is, simple scratching of the skin will suffice, without the use of histamine; in either case, the flare will stop abruptly at the border of the involved area. Unhappily, as Pardo-Castello has noted, the flare is hard to see against the pigmented background of a dark skin and almost impossible to identify in very deeply pigmented persons.

Easily read in such skins is the methacholine sweating test. Approximately 0.1 cc of a 1% solution of methacholine (Mecholyl®) chloride is injected intradermally either at the border of the lesion or both inside and outside, after painting the area with Minor's solution (2% iodine and 10% castor oil in absolute alcohol), and the area is then dusted with powdered starch, most easily applied with a powder-blower. Each secreted sweat droplet then moistens the dry iodine-starch combination and turns it deep blue.

Jeanselme, Degotte, and others have shown that pilocarpine will not stimulate the denervated sweat glands in leprous skin lesions; neither will methacholine, despite the fact that in high concentrations it acts, like pilocarpine, directly on the cells. Anhidrosis, as demonstrated in this way, may be an earlier manifestation of nerve damage than the occurrence of thermal anesthesia.

For practical purposes, however, it constitutes a rather shaky foundation for so serious a diagnosis as leprosy, and it should be used primarily for excluding that diagnosis in patients presenting only one or two hypopigmented macules. It cannot be relied on in the examination of face lesions, apparently; false "positive" anhidrosis reactions occur in that area, and the lesions of pityriasis simplex may show failure of sweat response, as may also the café au lait macules of neurofibromatosis. Mechanical obstruction of sweat ducts may also interfere with it, as in psoriasis, lichen simplex chronicus, miliaria, tropical anhidrosis, and probably, porokeratosis.

Chapter Six

CLINICAL PATTERN

LEPROMATOUS LEPROSY

L EPROMATOUS leprosy is the progressive—once called the "malignant"—form of the disease. It may well be thought of as a process in which the human host stores the leprosy bacilli in histiocytes in the skin, lymph nodes, liver, spleen, and bone marrow—and also, interestingly, in the more superficially situated nerves and in the testes. Mitsuda has described lepromatous infiltrates in the heart, stomach, intestine, kidney, bladder, and ovary, but these appear to be exceptional observations.

The histiocytes appear to be able to kill and destroy the bacilli only very slowly. It is a deficiency of cellular immunity, which will be discussed under immunology.

It is noteworthy that only in exceptional, and advanced cases, does the involvement of histiocytes in the internal viscera become clinically apparent, whereas the skin is involved early and conspicuously. It is also of interest that involvement of the eye is pretty well limited to the anterior portion: conjunctiva, cornea, anterior sclera, iris, and ciliary body. Further, mucous membrane involvement, a regular occurrence in these patients, is confined largely to the respiratory passages from the larynx, or sometimes the major bronchi, outward. Finally, the only "internal" organ regularly clinically damaged in lepromatous leprosy is the testis.

All of these tissues have a normal temperature below 98.6°F. It would appear that a temperature below the normal body temperature level facilitates the growth of the bacillus.

Clinical Features

Skin Lesions

The skin lesions of lepromatous leprosy present a most variegated clinical spectrum, and it is to the credit of leprologists that

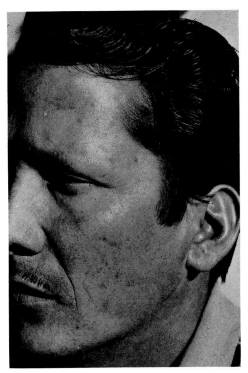

FIGURE 10. The face in diffuse lepromatosis. Note absence of eyebrows and lashes, and absence of disfiguring changes.

no elaborate classification of them has ever been developed. They do fall, however, into three general categories: macular, nodular, and the rare (except in Central America) pure diffuse or "spotted" leprosy of Lucio (Plate 6, Figs. 10, 11, and 12).

Macules of lepromatous leprosy are often hypopigmented (never completely depigmented) (Plate 1B), not very sharply defined at the borders, and more often multiple and widespread than solitary. They tend to be confluent. They may be erythematous, or bluish, and may be exanthematic (Plate 1A). They are frequently slightly infiltrated. They are usually smooth. They seldom manifest anesthesia or even anhidrosis, unlike the hypopigmented macule of tuberculoid leprosy.

Nodular lepromatous leprosy is the classic and most common variety. It is characterized by papular or nodular lesions (Figs.

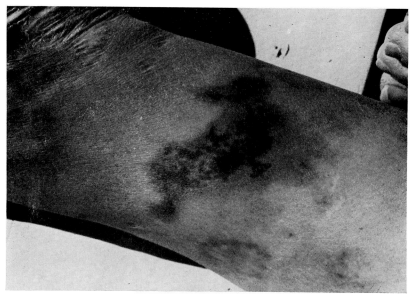

FIGURE 11. Erythema necroticans in diffuse lepromatosis (Lucio's phenomenon): bizarre-shaped dark-red macule with beginning ischemic necrosis and eschar formation. A stage between pictures A and B in Plate 6.

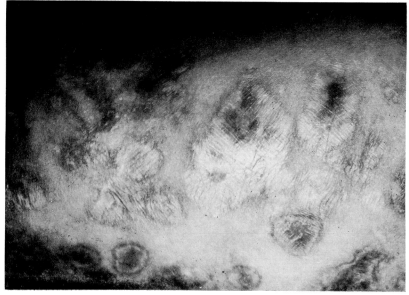

FIGURE 12. Diffuse lepromatosis: the ultimate scars, suggesting artefacts, resulting from erythema necroticans.

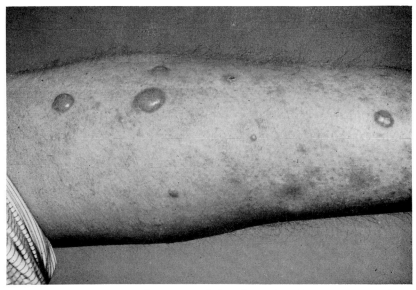

FIGURE 13. Lepromatous leprosy: nodules of varying size, on an arm, simulating dermatofibromas.

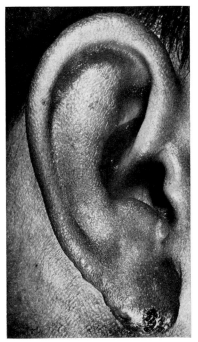

FIGURE 14. Lepromatous leprosy of helix and lobe of external ear, with a small crusted erosion.

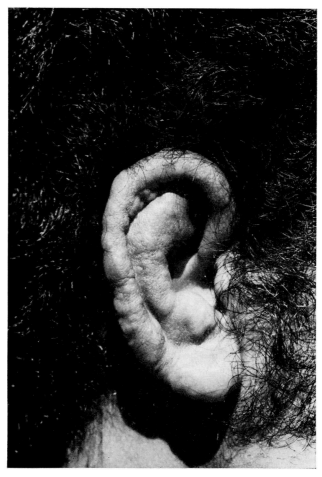

Figure 15. Lepromatous leprosy extensively involving the ear, a characteristic acral location for such lesions.

13-17), or plaques, which are often dull red, moderately elevated, often sharply defined (Plates 3 and 4) fixed in the dermis, and rarely ulcerated (Fig. 18) except, superficially, during lepra reactions. Their clinical resemblance to corresponding forms of lymphoma or leukemia (especially monocytic) of the skin is astonishingly exact (Plate 4), though this is not so surprising when one considers that lesions of both diseases are composed of histiocytic cells.

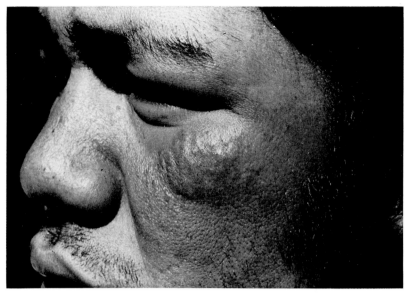

FIGURE 16. Lepromatous leprosy: a reactional flare-up of existing lesions, with characteristic erythema and edema.

The distribution and appearance of lepromas, as the nodular skin lesions of lepromatous leprosy are called, can be understood best if they are looked upon as a sort of foreign body granuloma in which the foreign bodies—the bacilli—grow and multiply; they represent an effective phagocytic process, but a rather ineffective defensive one; and as has been pointed out, they develop best in cool areas of skin.

They tend to avoid, then, areas where the subcutaneous tissue is scanty and dense—the scalp, the palms and soles, the intermammary fold, and the areas between the nasion and the internal ocular canthi. They also avoid the warmer areas, such as the axillae and groins, and the midline of the back, and involve by predilection the acral parts: the helices and lobes of the ears (Plate 2A, Figs. 14 and 15), the nose, lips and chin; the elbows, buttocks and knees. Their growth is so passive that the warmth and light pressure produced by wrinkling the skin, as on the forehead, tends to prevent their formation in the wrinkles: hence the deeply furrowed "leonine" facies of the advanced case (Fig.

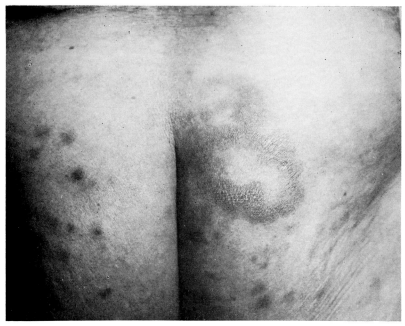

FIGURE 17. Borderline leprosy with two kinds of lesions: an annular plaque, with characteristic "inverted saucer" configuration (sharp, steep inner edge and indistinct, sloping outer edge) and intradermal nodules on the arm and back. Very few bacilli were present. Subsequent course marked by relapses even during maintenance therapy.

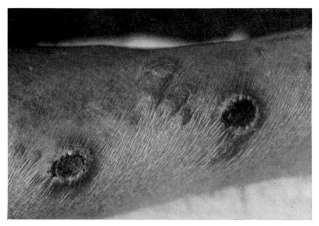

FIGURE 18. Lepromatous leprosy: crater-like vacciniform nodules on the arm, an exceptional picture, illustrative of leprosy's mimicry.

19). They are red, often with a peculiar brownish or coppery hue.

If a lepromatous plaque has an annular shape, as often happens, the inner margin is regularly steep and the outer one gently sloping, in contrast to the margins of tuberculoid plaques (Plate 2B, Fig. 17).

Nerve involvement is not an essential clinical feature of the leproma, and the skin covering these lesions may or may not be anesthetic. If it is anesthetic, the area of anesthesia—in contrast to that in tuberculoid leprosy—is independent of the skin lesion and usually extends beyond it.

Pure diffuse lepromatous leprosy, or spotted leprosy of Lucio, is a special form of the disease which is rare outside of Costa Rica and the State of Sinaloa, in Mexico, where it comprises from 30 to 60 percent of cases of lepromatous type. One probable example has been reported from Hawaii, one from Los Angeles by Obermayer, and one from New Orleans by Derbes. Originally

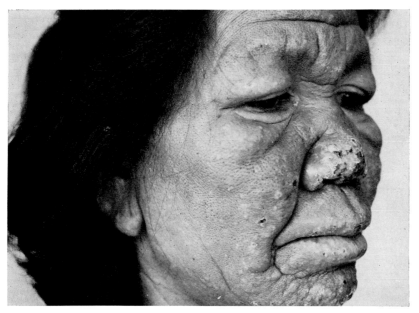

FIGURE 19. Lepromatous leprosy: note loss of brows and lashes, and deep furrowing, exaggerating the normal folds of the face. Involvement of supraorbital ridges, nose, lips, chin, and earlobes is characteristic.

described by Lucio and Alvarado in 1852, and known in Mexico in 1886 under the common name *lepra lazarina* as a distinct variety of the disease, it was long forgotten when in 1946 Latapi and Chevez Zamora, of Mexico, and in 1948 Obermayer, of Los Angeles, reminded us of it by a series of publications.

Two essential features distinguish it from ordinary lepromatous leprosy: first, none of the universal lepromatous infiltrate is circumscribed—no lepromas occur at any stage of the disease. Second, during reactive phases, crops of erythematous macules of irregular polygonal shape (Plate 6, Fig. 11) do occur ("erythema necroticans"), sometimes after formation of a flaccid bulla. They leave scars, so oddly shaped and atrophic as to suggest chemical burns or similar artefacts (Fig. 12).

It is a singularly rapidly progressive and malignant form of leprosy, terminating fatally (if not treated) in an average of only seven years. On inspection, during reactions, one sees only the bullae, eschars, ulcers, and scars on the legs and arms; loss of the eyebrows and, soon afterward, of all body hair, including eyelashes; and telangiectases on the cheeks. Between reactions, one sees only the hair loss. The cutaneous infiltration, though it involves every portion of the skin and renders it somewhat smooth and stiff, does not conspicuously distort or disfigure it and may easily entirely escape—as it did Lucio himself—the inexperienced examiner (Fig. 10). Because of this, Latapi has suggested the name *lepra bonita*: "pretty leprosy." Despite the absence of "lesions" in these cases, biopsy of the normal looking skin, in any site, will show abundant bacilli.

The word *lazarine*, though long usage justifies its application to this form of leprosy, has been given up, since it has also been applied to other bullous or ulcerative lesions of the disease.

Mucous Membrane Lesions

The nasal mucous membrane is often involved in lepromatous cases; ulceration and perforation or destruction of the cartilaginous septum occur commonly, with severe resultant nasal deformity in advanced cases.

Nasopharyngeal, pharyngeal, and palatal ulceration may occur,

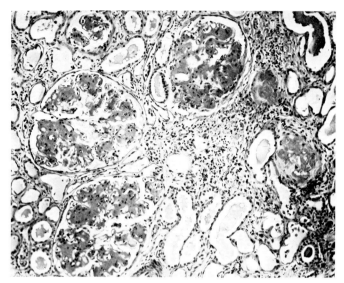

Figure 20. Amyloidosis of renal glomeruli in lepromatous leprosy. (Courtesy Irvin L. Tilden, M.D.)

the indirect evidence of liver damage mentioned above, and undoubtedly explains many of the deaths attributed to chronic nephritis.

Eye Lesions

The eye is regularly involved in advanced cases of lepromatous leprosy, except, as has been stated, in the pure diffuse type of Lucio. Involvement may be (a) infrequently, by direct extension; (b) most often, by hematogenous implantation of bacilli in the iris and ciliary body (Plate 8A) or (c) by eyelid paralysis (Fig. 3) due to nerve involvement, resulting in exposure keratitis. A lepromatous pannus may form on the eyeball and extend across the cornea. Glaucoma is an infrequent complication, except in cases of acute iritis. Eventual blindness is common, though by no means invariable, in untreated lepromatous leprosy.

Course

The course of untreated lepromatous leprosy in presulfone days was in general a progressive downhill one, with eventual fatal termination either from intercurrent tuberculosis (in roughly half of most series of cases) or amyloid nephrosis (in about one-sixth) or other causes. The disease itself is seldom a direct cause of death, except perhaps by producing laryngeal obstruction, but it so enfeebles the patient in advanced cases that other infections may have a fatal outcome. In Culion, according to Wade, it was quite common in the pre-sulfone era to see repeated reactions eventuate in fatal "cachexia leprosa." Exceptionally, and inexplicably, the disease may undergo gradual spontaneous regression and healing, producing "the burned-out case."

Under sulfone treatment, however, this has been radically changed. Adequate doses of dapsone prevent further progression of the disease in most cases, and in a substantial majority there is slow but steady regression of skin and mucosal lesions, early nerve lesions, and numbers of bacilli. The bacilli in treated cases become beaded and fragmented. Badly damaged nerves, however, rarely recover any appreciable degree of function.

Reactions

The commonest form of lepra reaction, occurring in about half of all lepromatous cases, usually after a year or two of treatment, is erythema nodosum leprosum (ENL). ENL may also occur in untreated patients and was the original reason for seeking medical advice in about 10% of patients seen at the USPHS Hospital in San Francisco. It was at one time thought to be a good sign, perhaps because it does not occur in patients still harboring live bacilli in the skin. The view that it is a favorable prognostic sign, however, is no longer held by most workers, ourselves included.

ENL begins with the appearance of crops of bright red, tender nodules from 1 to 2 or even 3 cm in diameter, on the extremities and face for the most part. Their configuration sometimes suggests erythema multiforme; they may even be bullous. They may become confluent, forming plaques. As they involute they may acquire a bluish color. Their distribution is unrelated to the existing leprous lesions. Fever and malaise often accompany them, and recurrent attacks may be increasingly severe. Painful swelling of peripheral nerves, notably the ulnar nerves, may accompany attacks, and may require surgical decortication.

Another manifestation of the lepra reaction, independent of ENL, is exacerbation of existing lepromatous lesions, and sometimes shallow ulceration of them, accompanied by appearance of new lesions and an increase in the number of bacilli in the tissue. Such an increase of bacilli is not noted in ENL reactions.

TUBERCULOID LEPROSY

Tuberculoid leprosy is the relatively benign, generally self-limited form of the disease, in which the host reacts defensively, and often successfully, against the invading bacillus. The defensive response has three major aspects: limitation of the disease to one or more circumscribed portions of the body; destruction of the bacilli; and eventual eradication of the infection. The defense depends on the patient's ability to manifest cellular immunity, as opposed to ineffective humoral immunity.

The term "tuberculoid" applied by Jadassohn to this type of leprosy in 1898 but only officially adopted in classification of the disease at the Havana Congress in 1948, is not wholly satisfactory, for it suggests that a tuberculoid histologic structure is an essential feature, and this is not the case. The word "tuberculoid" is used in two senses—in its original histologic sense of "resembling tuberculosis," to describe the noncaseating epithelioid-cell tubercles which characterize fully developed lesions of the disease; and also in the clinical sense of a relatively benign biologic type of leprosy. Hence it is conceivable that a relatively early case of tuberculoid leprosy might not yet present a tuberculoid histologic structure—though most cases do, as Wade and others have shown.

Most leprosy workers today apply the name "tuberculoid" type to all cases presenting lesions with foci of epithelioid cells, nerve involvement, a positive lepromin reaction, and no bacilli—even those showing only hypopigmented anesthetic or anhidrotic macules. We do, too.

Clinical Features

Skin Lesions

The skin lesions of tuberculoid leprosy are as protean as those of cutaneous tuberculosis or syphilis; indeed, Unna called them "leprides." Some examples of their mimicry have been recounted above. Proficiency in their diagnosis can only be acquired, as with skin lesions of any other disease, by seeing examples of them. Nevertheless, there may be some profit in describing them here.

Simple, flat, hypopigmented (*never* depigmented!) macules (Fig. 21) are decidedly more common in tuberculoid leprosy than in lepromatous, so much so that the term "macule" at one time signified, to leprologists, any circumscribed skin lesion, whether flat or elevated, of this form of the disease. It is for this reason that terms like "simple" and "flat" have come to be used to designate tuberculoid lesions which are macules in the stricter, dermatologic sense.

Macules of tuberculoid leprosy tend to be much less numerous than those of lepromatous, much more sharply defined, more discrete, and more often in exposed areas (Fig. 22), though the back and buttocks are also a site of election. Loss of sensation is an inconstant feature of these early lesions, especially on the face, but virtually all of them will show anhidrosis.

Tuberculoid plaques vary from aggregations of close-set, discrete papules (Fig. 1) giving a pebbled appearance to the in-

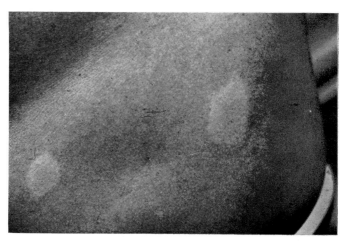

FIGURE 21. Tuberculoid leprosy: hypopigmented macules, anesthetic to cold and in part to light touch, on the back. Note sharp border. Easily confused with tinea versicolor or seborrheic dermatitis.

volved area ("minor tuberculoid" lesions), to sharply elevated, deep red, heavily infiltrated plaques ("major tuberculoid" lesions) (Fig. 23), which are often as much as 20 to 40 cm across. Central clearing is not unusual. Intermittent extension, alternating with periods of subsidence of activity, often produces "cockade" lesions of "borderline" leprosy with two, three, four, or more concentric annules (Fig. 24 and Plate 15B).

The appearance of sarcoid may be imitated quite exactly by

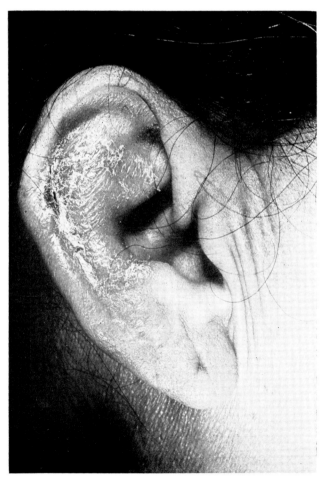

FIGURE 22. Tuberculoid leprosy: erythematous lesion, superficial scales, right external ear, resembling seborrheic dermatitis.

tuberculoid leprosy of the skin, though it is curious—and helpful, too—that the hyperglobulinemia and eye lesions which may be associated with the former are limited, in leprosy, to the lepromatous form. The most reliable clinical diagnostic point about tuberculoid plaques, minor or major, is their invariable association with anesthesia of the involved skin. The rarity or absence of acid-fast bacilli is also a regular feature of such lesions, except during reactions. Tuberculoid leprosy spares mucous membranes entirely: the nose, eyes, and respiratory passages are not involved.

Nerve Lesions

Nerve involvement is usually the most conspicuous feature of tuberculoid leprosy; hence the older names "neural" and "neuro-

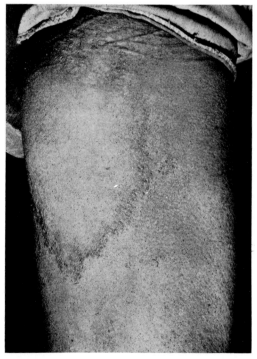

FIGURE 23. Major tuberculoid leprosy: annular plaque with irregular border on back of thigh. Note sharp outer margin, sloping inner one. The lesion was anesthetic to touch as well as temperature.

macular," still employed in India. The reason for this is a simple one: it is because a vigorous inflammatory defensive reaction occurs very early in the course of the disease, and the nerves—instead of serving largely as a repository for bacilli, as in the lepromatous case (see Fig. 14)—become a battleground. They suffer the usual fate of battlegrounds: severe damage.

The tendency in tuberculoid cases for the infection to be restricted to a comparatively limited area results, in many instances, in severe involvement of a single nerve; thus, only one great auricular nerve may be markedly swollen (Fig. 8) or only one hand contracted by ulnar neuritis, or only one toe rendered anesthetic by involvement of a single branch of the sural nerve. In other cases an area of anesthesia may occur in otherwise normal skin, as a result of tuberculoid leprous neuritis of underlying nerves.

The loss of nerve function is frequently only partial, usually beginning with sympathetic (sudomotor, pilomotor, and vasomotor) nerves and progressing to involve, often separately and successively, fibers mediating sensations of touch, heat, cold, and pain. Pressure and vibratory senses, and deep tendon reflexes, are lost only very late, if at all. Motor fibers are destroyed gradually, so that muscular weakness and loss of muscle tone occur before actual paralysis and muscular atrophy. Contracture of unparalyzed opposing muscles, notably in the hands (Fig. 7), occurs regularly in advanced cases, though it is inconspicuous and without significance if much absorption of bone occurs as well.

Trophic disturbances also result from nerve damage, and it must be understood that these, like other consequences of neuritis, occur in both lepromatous and tuberculoid cases. Trophic changes take three principal forms: a dry brown scaliness and atrophy of the skin, especially on the lower legs; perforating ulcers, usually of the soles; and concentric absorption of bone, usually limited largely to the phalanges (of both hands and feet) and metatarsals (Figs. 9 and 25).

Perforating ulcers have been mentioned under diagnosis (Chapter 5). They frequently lead to osteomyelitis, which must be treated on its own account if the ulcer is to be made to heal.

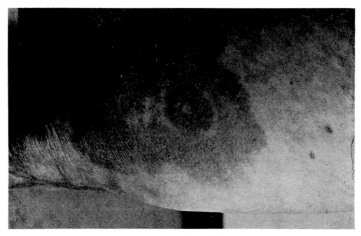

FIGURE 24. Borderline leprosy: a "cockade" lesion with four zones of alternating activity and normal looking skin.

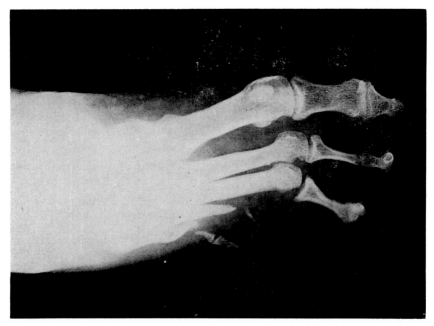

FIGURE 25. Concentric trophic absorption of bone in late leprosy of nerves: distal phalanges have disappeared from all but the great toe, and the remaining ones, as well as the fourth and fifth metatarsals, show thinning and ultimate breaking of the shafts.

A great deal of disability in advanced but "burned out" old cases of leprosy is caused by these ulcers.

Concentric absorption and thinning of the shafts of the phalanges and metatarsals (but only very rarely the metacarpals) is a characteristic feature of advanced leprosy of nerves. When the shaft finally thins to the breaking point, the surrounding soft tissues contract and the digits are shortened. "Dropping off" of digits never occurs, and a hand which has lost all of its fingers will often be seen to have retained remnants, at least, of finger-nails (Fig. 9). Loss of vasomotor tone produces characteristic diffuse cyanosis and puffiness of the hands and feet and sometimes of the trunk as well.

Visceral Lesions

The internal organs, including the testicle, are not involved in tuberculoid leprosy. Epithelioid-cell tubercles have rarely been seen in lymph nodes.

The hyperglobulinemia, biologic false positive serologic tests for syphilis, elevated sedimentation rate, and so forth, that occur so regularly in the lepromatous case, do not occur, for practical purposes, in the tuberculoid. This fact has been used from time to time as an aid in differentiating the two types, though other criteria are much more reliable. The visceral amyloidosis seen so frequently in advanced lepromatous cases at autopsy does not occur in tuberculoid cases, apparently, though of course autopsy material is far less abundant in the latter.

Eye Lesions

Damage to the cornea through exposure by reason of paralysis of the eyelids may complicate a case of tuberculoid leprosy. Even this is not common, and actual primary leprous involvement of the eye does not occur in the tuberculoid form of the disease.

Course

The course of the tuberculoid case, untreated (and treated as well, in some instances), is paradoxical. In general it is benign, with spontaneous regression and healing of the lesion, or lesions, often within a year or so of the onset; but so rapid and complete may be the destruction of involved nerves that in some instances the patient is worse off than if he had been a lepromatous case.

Tuberculoid Reactions

Like the lepromatous case, the tuberculoid case may undergo intermittent episodes of exacerbation. Lesions become more inflamed, edematous, elevated, reddened, often painful, and hypersensitive; one or more involved nerves may become acutely swollen and painful or even abscessed; bacilli in considerable numbers may appear in the tissues; exceptionally, low-grade fever may occur. Erythema multiforme does not appear, however.

In tuberculoid leprosy, reactions consist either in a flare-up of existing lesions with appearance of bacilli in them ("tuberculoid reactivation"), without systemic symptoms, or in a more severe form characterized by sudden appearance of fresh lesions, sometimes concentric with existing lesions, forming a "cockade" pattern, with fairly numerous bacilli ("reactional tuberculoid leprosy"). Fever is absent or very slight, and ENL and erythema multiforme do not occur.

BORDERLINE LEPROSY

In Danielssen's anatomical classification of leprosy, virtually all cases were "mixed" cases. In Hansen's biological classification, he regarded almost all cases as either "tubercular" (lepromatous) or "maculoanesthetic" (tuberculoid) and thus, as he said, "we delete altogether the title of 'mixed' leprosy."

During the thirties and forties, Windsor Wade published a series of papers in which he developed the concept of "borderline" leprosy: cases on the borderline, so to speak, between tuberculoid and lepromatous types. Khanolkar and Cochrane, during the fifties, proposed the name "dimorphous" for this group of cases and attempted to extend the concept to include the indeterminate (originally *incaracteristico*) cases described by the Latin American leprologists, in which there is not so much evidence of both types of leprosy, as evidence of neither one.

"Borderline" leprosy, as this form is now generally called in preference to "dimorphous," has as a rule rather more of the characteristics of tuberculoid leprosy than of lepromatous. It may be either unilateral and asymmetric, or bilateral; it is not often symmetrical, however. Mucous membrane lesions and eye lesions are not seen. Eyebrows are not lost. ENL does not occur; reactions consist of exacerbation of leprous lesions. Nerve involvement is often early and severe, and anesthesia and motor weakness are usually present. Bacilli are always present but in small numbers. The lepromin test is either weakly positive or negative.

The skin lesions are usually elevated, red plaques, often annular, with steep inner borders and gently sloping periphery, like an inverted saucer (Plate 10, Fig. 2). "Cockade" lesions (Fig. 24, Plate 15B) are often seen. Macular lesions may occur. Histologically, both tuberculoid and lepromatous features are seen, sometimes in different portions of a lesion, sometimes mixed together. This will be discussed under histopathology.

Borderline leprosy is either actually or potentially in transition toward either the lepromatous type or the tuberculoid type. Because of this, the symbols "BB," "BL," and "BT," have been developed. (See Table III.)

In "BB" leprosy, the situation is rather in the middle of the road, with little evidence of instability or of progression toward either polar type. In a "BL" case, bacilli are numerous, the lepromin reaction is negative, and the clinical features may suggest activity and aggression. Such a patient is likely to become lepromatous fairly soon, if not treated, with frequent reactional flares. In a "BT" case, on the other hand, the lepromin reaction is at least weakly positive, perhaps even one or two plus; bacilli are present though not numerous; lesions are asymmetric and not extensive. In such a case the prognosis is good for eventual conversion to tuberculoid type, even without treatment, though of course all such cases should be treated.

INDETERMINATE LEPROSY

The basic lesion is a pale, slightly hypopigmented, occasionally faint pink macule, round or oval. Its size varies between 1 and 3 cm. The surface is smooth, the margins not well demarcated.

There is no infiltration. The lesion is asymptomatic, usually not anesthetic. It is usually single, but can occur in small numbers. Lesions of indeterminate leprosy are located on the trunk, upper extremities, or on the face.

The clinical manifestations of indeterminate leprosy can easily escape attention. It is most often diagnosed in contacts where the index of suspicion is high.

"HANSEN'S DISEASE" VERSUS "LEPROSY"

Because of the connotation of fear of contagion and opprobrium, that have come to be attached to the word "leprosy," there has for many years been a movement to officially abandon it in favor of the eponym "Hansen's disease," or even "hanseniasis." Patients at Carville leprosarium, especially the late Stanley Stein, Editor of the Carville *Star* and coauthor of *Alone No Longer,* have been the principal proponents of the change. They argue that the word "leprosy" was originally, and may still properly be, used to mean "a scaly disease"; that it is used in this sense in the Bible; and that fear of contagiousness, and a feeling of shame, are so firmly attached to the name, rather than to the disease itself, that patients are made to suffer unnecessarily by retaining this name for the disease.

At the Havana Congress, in 1948, a special committee under the sympathetic chairmanship of Mr. Perry Burgess* was appointed to consider this proposal. Numerous hearings and discussions were held, and a recommendation was made that "leprosy" should be retained as the official designation for the disease, though "leper" should be abandoned entirely as the designation for a leprous patient. The Congress approved the committee's recommendations. With this view we strongly agree.

---

* Mr. Burgess was President of the Leonard Wood Memorial Foundation and the author of *Who Walk Alone* and *Born of Those Years.* He died in 1958.

Chapter Seven

IMMUNOLOGY

A RMAUER HANSEN threw the first light on the immunologic aspects of leprosy in 1895 by distinguishing between two *biologic* types—lepromatous and tuberculoid—instead of merely separating two *anatomical* types—cutaneous and neural—as Danielsson had done. In lepromatous leprosy, low resistance and steady progression of disease were the almost invariable rule; in tuberculoid, high resistance and sometimes a short stormy course toward spontaneous recovery, except for residual nerve damage.

Kensuke Mitsuda at Aiseien in Japan, some twenty years later, reported that patients with lepromatous leprosy showed no skin reaction to an intracutaneous injection of "lepromin"—a ground-up mixture of autoclaved *M leprae* and tissue elements, suspended in saline. Tuberculoid leprosy patients, however, always manifested a strong skin reaction, requiring about three weeks to become full blown (Fig. 26).

Dharmendra, about twenty-five years after Mitsuda, broke down Mitsuda's lepromin by separating the bacilli from the tissue elements and fractionating them and elicited the reaction in seventy-two hours. This confirmed what had already been suspected: that the reaction showed delayed skin sensitivity to the organism. His test material has been referred to as leprolin. Little or no increase in either sensitivity or specificity was achieved by this, however, so the method, a tedious and difficult one, never became popular.

Histologically, the positive reaction closely resembles active tuberculoid leprosy; the negative one shows only banal lymphocytic infiltration in addition to the injected bacilli. Wade was able to completely block the reaction by the simultaneous or prior injection of hydrocortisone.

It must be emphasized that *the lepromin reaction is not a diagnostic test for leprosy*; many nonleprous persons have a posi-

63

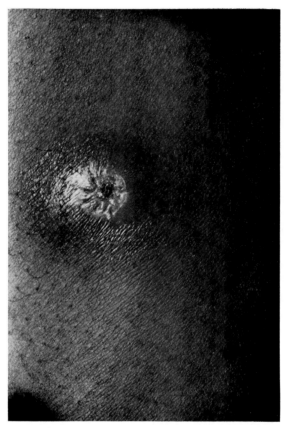

FIGURE 26. Strongly positive lepromin (Mitsuda) reaction, three weeks after injection: an edematous, reddened papule measuring about 8 x 10 mm.

tive lepromin reaction; dogs frequently give a positive response; and surveys of populations in relatively leprosy-free areas such as New York and Paris have shown as high as 75 percent of the population to give a positive response, although Cochrane and Dielding found only 3 percent positive reactors among three hundred medical students in Australia.

In summary, a negative lepromin reaction in persons who presumably do not have leprosy might suggest lack of capacity for cellular immunity against the infection. In persons who do have leprosy, the negative test is characteristic of the lepromatous type. In other than frankly lepromatous leprosy, it suggests that the disease may be on its way to becoming lepromatous, and is therefore a bad prognostic sign.

A positive lepromin reaction does not mean that the patient has leprosy; but if leprosy *is* present, such a reaction suggests that it is of tuberculoid type or, if it is not of tuberculoid type, that it may be on its way to becoming so; it is therefore a good prognostic sign.

A weakly positive reaction—a papule less than 5 mm in diameter—is of course inconclusive, and must be interpreted, if it can be interpreted at all, in the light of all the other facts in the case.

As our sophistication in immunology has increased, additional evidence has enabled us to contrast the two polar types of leprosy. In reacting tuberculoid lesions, we find the characteristics of delayed hypersensitivity, as the positive skin test has already led us to expect: abundant lymphocytes; low titers of anti-mycobacterial antibody; few organisms; and no, or very few, plasma cells. In lepromatous granulomatous tissue, on the contrary, we find macrophages full of organisms, and in reacting lesions, such as those of erythema nodosum leprosum, we see a vasculitis like that of serum sickness, with some plasma cells and few lymphocytes. It has also been shown that serum complement is used up, presumably by antigen-antibody binding, in such lesions.

The determining factor in deciding which of these two patterns will occur in a given patient may be genetic: either racial, or familial. Lepromatous leprosy among the Burmese in Assam, for example, is twice as common as tuberculoid, while the reverse is true among Indians in that country. Chinese in Africa, similarly, have far more lepromatous leprosy than tuberculoid, while the ratio is reversed among Africans. A given family, moreover, will often be observed to have all lepromatous cases, or, much more rarely (the transmissibility being so low), all tuberculoid. There is reason to believe that racial immunity may be acquired through long endemicity of the disease.

The differences do not stop with histopathology, however. As shown by Bullock, lepromatous patients have a generalized impairment of their capacity to express delayed hypersensitivity as measured by skin tests with non-mycobacterial antigens. It is also difficult to establish *de novo* contact sensitization with haptens such as picryl chloride.

In vitro studies show that lymphocyte DNA synthesis in response to various stimulants is also abnormal. ^{3}H-thymidine uptake in response to phytohemagglutinin (PHA) may be severely decreased in lymphocytes from patients with lepromatous leprosy, as is the response to various antigens such as streptolysin O.

Recent studies by Bullock and Fasal have demonstrated the presence of an inhibitory substance in lepromatous serum that suppresses response to antigens *in vitro*; when lepromatous cells are washed and cultured in normal homologous serum, their response to antigens is improved. The poor response to PHA is not improved, however, thus suggesting that both an intrinsic defect of lymphocytes and a circulating immuno-inhibitory factor may be present in many of these patients.

The migration of guinea pig macrophages is strongly inhibited by a combination of lepromin with lymphocytes from a tuberculoid case, but only very weakly depressed if lymphocytes from a lepromatous patient are used. Thus, lepromatous lymphocytes appear to be defective in release of macrophage inhibitory factor when exposed to lepromin. Finally, skin allografts are rejected relatively slowly by lepromatous patients, but with almost normal rapidity by tuberculoid.

The macrophages themselves, however, in lepromatous patients, may also be specifically defective, as Olaf Skinsnes suggests. The bacillus-loaded macrophage in a lepromatous lesion does show lysosomal activity under the electron microscope: bacilli are being slowly digested. We cannot compare this with the situation in tuberculoid granulomatous tissue, however, because there we find few or no bacilli, so swiftly are they decapsulated and destroyed. So efficient is this process, even in the relatively ineffective macrophages of untreated lepromatous patients, that most of the bacilli are nonviable, though still not destroyed. Their lipid remains in the cell, and even after disappearance of many or most of the organisms, it is still valid diagnostically as a histologic marker of the lepromatous lesion. It is not retained in any significant amount in the histiocytes of tuberculoid lesions.

Skinsnes hypothesizes that a defect in the ability of the tissue macrophages to digest a lipid component of the bacilli is the major deficiency. Neutral fat and fatty acids are both increased in older foam cells. We have known since Unna that their vacuoles contain fat, and that by far the greater part of it is from the bacilli—not the tissue, as Mitsuda thought. Hansen's first stain for the organisms (luckily, since he picked it at random) was 1% osmic acid, which stains their fatty capsule pretty well. It has been just lucky, again, that the Ziehl-Neelsen carbol-fuchsin stain has worked as well as it has, since it tends to decapsulate the bacilli by the actions of both phenol and heat.

Bullock *et al.* have attempted to confer the missing resistance upon lepromatous patients, by administering transfer factor from tuberculoid patients or from normal persons with a strongly positive lepromin reaction. In six of nine patients so treated, these investigators were able to achieve transfer of weak reactivity to lepromin. Furthermore, the patients experienced reactional changes within their lesions, beginning a few days after transfer and lasting between seven and twelve days. Grossly, the reactive changes resembled those seen in the so-called reversal reaction, which occurs spontaneously in some patients on DDS therapy and is associated with a favorable prognosis.

In a long-term follow-up, Bullock and co-workers have unfortunately observed no permanent clinical improvement in patients treated with transfer factor. This work does suggest, however, that preliminary treatment with DDS to reduce total antigen load, followed by repeated, large doses of transfer factor, may well be of value in providing more lasting cell-mediated immunity against the leprosy bacillus. Hopefully, this will reduce the current high rates of relapse, which may, if treatment is stopped, approach 40%. Obviously, great caution is indicated, because the activation of immune inflammation within nerve lesions, for example, could threaten the integrity of remaining nerve function if not carefully controlled.

Chapter Eight

HISTOPATHOLOGY

THE SAME wide spectrum observed in the clinical manifestations of leprosy is found in its histopathology. Some features are characteristic (diagnostic), others uncharacteristic (not diagnostic).

One feature found in all types and forms of leprosy is nerve involvement: *M leprae* has a predilection for peripheral nerves. The changes in skin and nerves reflect in their pathology the immunological status of the patient.

Ridley's histopathological classification of leprosy is based on the two polar *types*—lepromatous (L) and tuberculoid (T)— and three borderline groups, ranging from lepromatous through borderline lepromatous (BL), borderline (B), and borderline tuberculoid (BT), to tuberculoid (Table III). For immunological research Ridley recommends the addition of two histologic subpolar groups, lepromatous indefinite (LI), and tuberculoid indefinite (TI).

Two main cell types can be distinguished: (a) the lepra cell, a macrophage seen in polar lepromatous leprosy and borderline lepromatous leprosy, and (b) the epithelioid cell, found in polar tuberculoid leprosy and also in borderline tuberculoid and borderline leprosy.

Another cell type is the lymphocyte, which is of great importance for its role in mediating immunity. In addition to their importance in polar tuberculoid leprosy and in borderline tuberculoid leprosy, they can be of significance in borderline lepromatous leprosy.

Lepromatous leprosy is characterized by the presence of macrophages (lepra cells, Virchow cells), foamy histiocytes (Fig. 27) with numerous *M leprae*, in untreated lepromatous leprosy. Although the ratio of solidly staining bacilli to beaded bacilli (the MI) declines during treatment, the total number of bacilli

TABLE III
FIVE-GROUP CLASSIFICATION OF LEPROSY
(Modified, after Ridley)

5 Group Classification	T	BT	B	BL	L
Lepromin reaction	3+	1+	—	—	—
Immunological stability	++	±	—	±	++
Borderline reactions	—	±	++	+	—
ENL	—	—	—	—	+
Bacilli in granuloma	0	1—3+	3—4+	4—5+	5—6+
Epithelioid cells	+	+	+	—	—
Langhans giant cells	+	++	—	—	—
Touton giant cells	—	—	—	—	+
Globi	—	—	—	—	+
Foam cells	—	—	—	+	+++
Lymphocytes	+++	++	+	+++/+	±
Erosion of epidermis	+	—	—	—	—
Infiltration subepid. zone	+	±/—	—	—	—
Nerve destruction (skin)	++	++	+	±	—

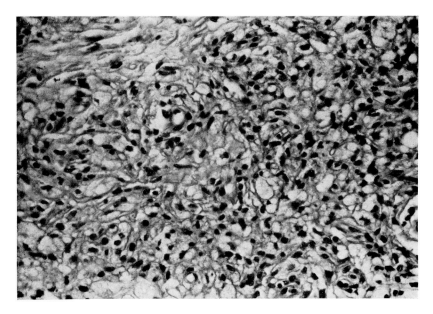

FIGURE 27.   Lepromatous leprosy: foam cells.

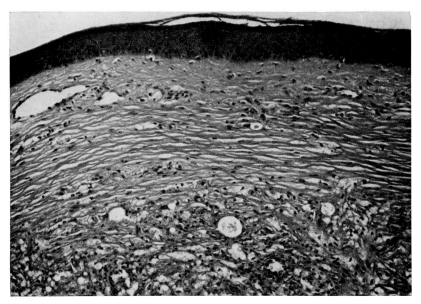

FIGURE 28. Lepromatous leprosy: wide zone of normal connective tissue between epidermis and granuloma. Large foam cells (lepra cell, Virchow cell).

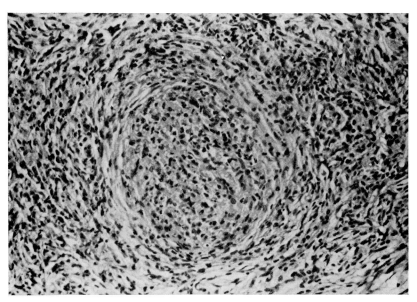

FIGURE 29. Lepromatous leprosy: cutaneous nerve surrounded and invaded by foam cells.

(the BI) may remain virtually unchanged, often for years. The bacilli can be found arranged in parallel formations (cigarette packs) or in globular masses (globi). They sometimes even show in hematoxylin-eosin stained sections as bluish shadows (Fig. 28).

Lepra cells can be present in small groups and strands, as observed in macular lesions, or in tumor-like masses, with all degrees in between these extremes (Fig. 27). The granuloma of lepromatous leprosy shows absence of focalization. It can replace or invade any and all structures of the skin. Although tumor-like formations can be found in the corium, they do not quite touch the epidermis. The granuloma in lepromatous leprosy is separated from the epidermis by a zone of normal connective tissue called the clear zone, or grenz zone. The width of this zone varies greatly. It can be so wide that it will be unlikely, when doing a snip (skin scraping), that the bacilli-containing granuloma can be reached (Fig. 28): one more argument for performing biopsies instead of skin scrapings in lepromatous leprosy!

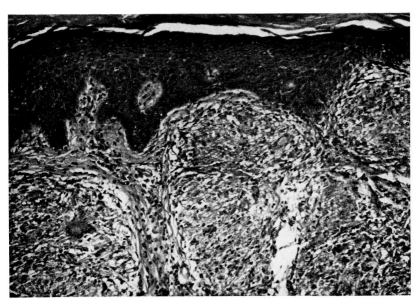

FIGURE 30. Tuberculoid leprosy: granuloma consisting of epithelioid cells, round cells, and Langhans' giant cells in upper corium, touching the epidermis.

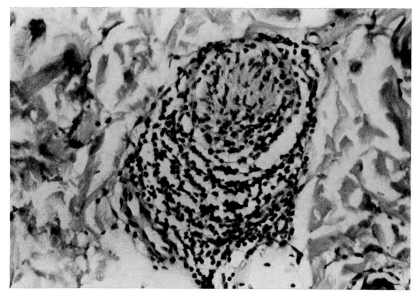

FIGURE 31. Tuberculoid leprosy: cutaneous nerve surrounded by round cells, showing slight degenerative changes.

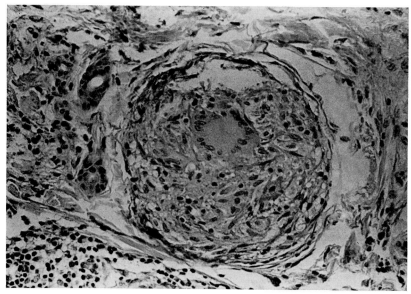

FIGURE 32. Tuberculoid leprosy: cutaneous nerve invaded by tuberculoid granuloma.

Nerves will contain bacilli, but foam cells invade them rather late. They are, however, usually surrounded by granuloma (Fig. 29).

In tuberculoid leprosy, the epithelioid cell is the characteristic cell. Its presence is evidence for host resistance. They are usually arranged in cords and may have an admixture of Langhans' giant cells (Fig. 30). The granuloma formed by epithelioid cells is not diagnostic for leprosy. It might mean sarcoid, tuberculosis, a tuberculid, a foreign body granuloma, or numerous other conditions. Lepra bacilli, which would be diagnostic, are frequently absent in tuberculoid leprosy, or only present in such small numbers that an extremely time-consuming search is necessary to find some. In sections, the most reliable diagnostic feature of tuberculoid leprosy is selective nerve involvement, which can vary in degree from a perineural infiltrate (Fig. 31) to invasion of the nerve by a tuberculoid granuloma (Fig. 32), leading to complete destruction.

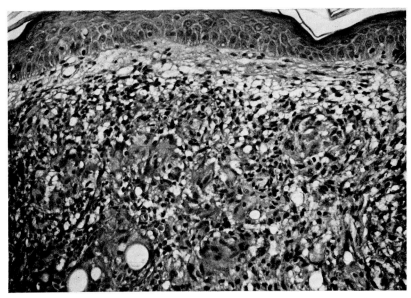

FIGURE 33. Borderline leprosy: narrow zone of connective tissue between epidermis and granuloma; granuloma consisting of foam cells, epithelioid cells and giant cells.

It is of the utmost importance that the nerve involvement is selective, independent of the granuloma, as nerves adjacent to a granuloma can be affected simply by continuity, a condition of course not diagnostic for leprosy.

In tuberculoid leprosy, the granuloma often touches the epidermis, and there is no free "grenz" zone as seen in lepromatous leprosy. Lymphocytes usually surround the epithelioid-cell granuloma in tuberculoid leprosy, in contrast to the so-called naked tubercles seen in sarcoid. The nerve involvement is early and rapid in tuberculoid leprosy, and late and slow in lepromatous leprosy.

In borderline leprosy, both cell types are present (Fig. 33), their ratio depending on the place in the spectrum: borderline lepromatous will show more lepra cells, borderline tuberculoid more epithelioid cells. The nerve involvement is most marked in borderline tuberculoid, often leading to caseation and necrosis.

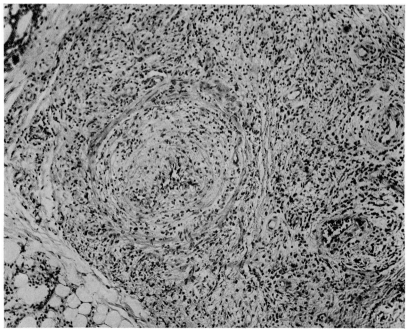

FIGURE 34. Blood vessel in erythema necroticans (diffuse lepromatosis): marked thickening of walls. Vessel surrounded and invaded by foam cells.

This explains the often serious, rapid, and severe clinical manifestations and complications.

Bacilli are present in borderline, borderline lepromatous, and lepromatous lesions, rare in borderline tuberculoid, and often absent in tuberculoid.

The most difficult diagnosis is indeterminate leprosy, as in many lesions of that group no characteristics of any type have yet developed. It begins with an inflammatory infiltrate consisting of round cells, around some of the blood vessels and skin appendages and also perineurally. If nerves are infiltrated, it is usually possible to find a few bacilli, enabling one to make a definite diagnosis. It does not appear advisable to make a diagnosis of indeterminate leprosy from the clinical appearance and contact history alone. It should always be substantiated by histopathological findings. However, if such a doubtful case has been in close contact with a patient with active lepromatous leprosy, he should be put on prophylactic treatment.

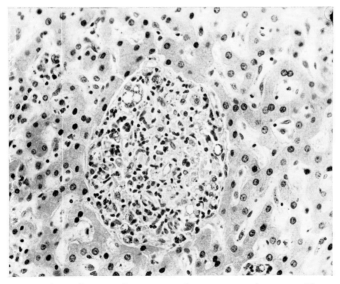

FIGURE 35. Miliary hepatic leproma in lepromatous leprosy. Note normal liver parenchyma: it is the reticuloendothelial (Kupffer) cells that are primarily involved. Vacuolated lepra cells of Virchow are well shown. Bacilli are numerous. (Courtesy Irvin L. Tilden, M.D.)

In erythema nodosum leprosum one usually finds foci of foam cells throughout the corium and subcutis, surrounded and invaded by round cells. Vasculitis of varying degrees is present.

A special form of lepromatous leprosy is the so-called diffuse lepromatosis, originally reported from the State of Sinaloa in Mexico. In these patients, one can find in normal appearing skin, which might show on H and E stain only a few perivascular round cells, innumerable acid-fast bacilli in the blood vessel walls and perivascularly. Even if there is no pathology in hematoxylin-eosin stained sections, acid-fast stains can give surprising results. If a patient with diffuse lepromatosis suffers a reaction—an equivalent of erythema nodosum leprosum in the lepromatous type—he will develop the so-called erythema necroticans, histologically a circumscribed infarct-like necrosis of the epidermis and corium with severe vascular involvement (Fig. 34). This is the so-called Lucio phenomenon.

Of internal organs, we find bacilli and granulomata, often only minute, in the liver (Fig. 35), spleen, and testicles. Foam cells

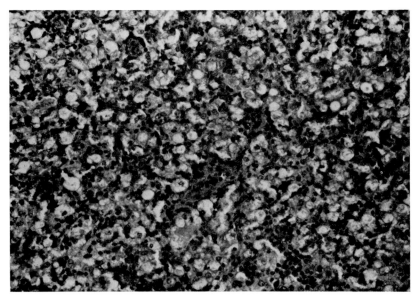

FIGURE 36. Lymph node in lepromatous leprosy. Invasion by foam cells destroying normal structure.

with large numbers of bacilli can be found in lymph nodes (Fig. 36), and sometimes in the bone marrow. Large numbers of bacilli, sometimes with severe destruction, are found in the eye (Plate 8A). Bacilli, without reactive changes, can be found even in the pulp of teeth.

Chapter Nine

TREATMENT

GENERAL PRINCIPLES

IT IS advisable to hospitalize all newly diagnosed cases of lepromatous leprosy for complete examination and initiation of chemotherapy. This is best done for cases with extensive involvement in a specialized center like the USPHS Hospital in Carville, the Hale Mohalu Hospital in Honolulu, or the Leprosy Service of the USPHS Hospital in San Francisco.

Most patients with tuberculoid leprosy can be handled without any hospitalization at all. For an early uncomplicated case of lepromatous leprosy, a short period in a general hospital might suffice, provided expert consultation is available. This avoids exposing the patient to the emotional shock of seeing himself as an "inmate" of a leprosy hospital.

Isolation is no longer regarded as vitally important, so rapidly does contagiousness decline under chemotherapy. The chief purpose of hospitalization is not for isolation, but rather to facilitate close observation during the sometimes difficult initial period of treatment in lepromatous cases.

HISTORICAL BACKGROUND

Chaulmoogra oil was used for leprosy in India both orally and externally as early as 500 B. C., but was not introduced into European medicine until 1854, when Dr. F. J. Mourat prepared the oil from the seeds. In 1919, Dean and Wrenshall in Hawaii prepared an iodized ethyl ester of the oil, a better-tolerated substance, marketed in 1922 under the name of Antileprol or "Dean's derivative." Its use resulted in a three or four fold increase of discharges from isolation, during the five or six years of its use, but relapses were prompt and numerous. Hansen himself gave up chaulmoogra oil as ineffective, but Victor Heiser in 1914 and Rogers in 1916 promoted a revival of interest in it.

Was it effective? Probably, at least occasionally, it was. There are innumerable glowing reports of successes achieved with it, based on observations by highly qualified and unquestionably honest observers. But its proponents steadily diminished in number, and by 1940 only three or four remained convinced that it was a useful drug. Still, sodium chaulmoograte has recently been shown by L. Levy and P. Jacobsen to be active against seventeen species of cultivable mycobacteria, and chaulmoogra may make a comeback yet!

SULFONES

Fromm and Whitman synthesized 4:4′ diamino diphenyl sulfone (DDS, or dapsone) in 1908, but it was nearly thirty years before its antibacterial activity was first investigated. It was then found to be highly toxic, inducing methemoglobinemia occasionally, hemolytic anemia often, and sometimes even serious bone marrow depression.

This led to the same approach used thirty years earlier with Ehrlich's first spirocheticidal compound, atoxyl: a search for substituted derivatives of lower toxicity. The first of these to be given a serious trial was glucosulfone sodium (Promin, Parke, Davis), which had proved disappointing against tuberculosis and was both literally and figuratively a "drug on the market." Guy Faget at the USPHS Hospital (then the U. S. Marine Hospital) in Carville, Louisiana, gave the drug intravenously to patients with lepromatous leprosy and established, in the initial trial, that it could produce striking clinical and bacteriological improvement in such cases.

A second derivative was sulphetrone, used chiefly in India and Africa by British workers; a third was Diasone® (Abbott), especially popular in Central America; another was Promacetin®. Though these compounds all had similar toxicity to the parent substance, they could be given in much larger doses without frequent or severe toxic effects.

Cochrane, in India, then tried the parent substance, dapsone, in very small doses—in the same way that oxophenarsine, so

nearly like Ehrlich's atoxyl, had been used a few years before—
and found that it was therapeutically effective in small, generally
subtoxic doses. Since then it has steadily grown in popularity
at the expense of its derivatives, and has now virtually completely replaced them.

Dapsone is available under that name in England, and in the
United States under the trade names Avlosulfon® and Novo-
phone®, in 10-, 25-, and 100-mg tablets. The dermatological
dose of 100 mg once or twice a day is far too high for lepromatous leprosy; it is not only unnecessary, but is likely to cause
severe toxic effects. The optimum dose in leprosy has never been
determined.

In tuberculoid leprosy, the drug is well tolerated, but a very
small dose is sufficient; 50 mg twice a week may be given from
the beginning and continued until clinical recovery is complete
and for a sufficient period afterward (say, at least two to five
years) to assure a permanent result.

In lepromatous leprosy, the drug is less well tolerated and full
doses are not advisable. Initial dosage must be small. At Carville the following schedule is used:

Week	Dose of DDS
1	25 mg twice
2	50 mg twice
3–6	100 mg twice a week
7–10	100 mg three times a week
11 ff	100 mg four times a week

The schedule at Hale Mohalu in Honolulu is as follows:

Week	25 mg, x/week
1	1
2	2
3	3
4	4
5	5
6	6
7 ff	Daily

Dharmendra, in India, suggests 25 mg once a week initially,
increased very slowly to 100 mg a day, 6 days a week. Pettit at
Sungei Buloh suggests 100 mg twice a week from the very be-

ginning, and not increasing the dose at all. Our own recommendation is to give the following doses:

Week	Dose of DDS
1 & 2	50 mg 2x/week*
3 ff	50 mg daily

Prior to Shepard's demonstration in 1960, through mouse footpad inoculation, that only solidly staining bacilli are viable and potentially infectious, treatment used to be moderated entirely through two parameters: (1) clinical improvement and (2) the reduction of the total number of bacilli. These two parameters do show improvement during treatment over a period of four to six years in almost all cases. It was customary in those years to require isolation of lepromatous cases until bacilli could no longer be found in smears or sections.

Our chief concern today, however, is not with the bacteriologic index (BI)—the number of bacilli per high power field—but with the morphologic index (MI): the percentage of bacilli which stain solidly from end to end and are therefore presumably alive. In cases responding favorably, the MI should drop from a maximum initial level (which may range anywhere from 10 to 80%, depending on the observer) to nearly zero by the third to sixth month of treatment with dapsone—or sooner with rifampin.

We must not forget that this observation applies only to bacilli in readily examined skin lesions. It is quite likely that viable organisms remain in other areas, especially in nerves. An MI of zero does not imply cure. Mouse footpad inoculation might still be positive. Treatment must be continued in lepromatous cases for life, although the dose of dapsone can and should be reduced to a maintenance level, perhaps 50 mg twice a week, after four or five years' treatment, depending on the clinical improvement and the decline of the BI. In Hawaii the relapse rate in treated lepromatous cases has reached 25% after five years without treatment, over a twenty-year period of observation.

A repository sulfone, diacetyl diamino diphenyl sulfone, called

---

* This dose is not increased in "borderline," or in tuberculoid, cases; 50 mg twice a week is sufficient for them.

diacetyl dapsone or DADDS, has been given some clinical field trials with impressive results in both chemoprophylaxis and treatment. A dose of 225 mg intramuscularly every seventy-five days releases dapsone into the circulation at a rate of about 2.4 mg a day. The clinical and bacteriologic response was found by Shepard *et al.* in a trial conducted in the Philippines, to be identical to that expected from oral dapsone. Toxicity is negligible. This observation has been confirmed in large trials by Russell *et al.* in New Guinea, and by Sloan *et al.* in Micronesia. DADDS shows great promise, but it may be that a somewhat larger dose (or more frequent doses) may be necessary.

The convenience and certainty of medication achieved in this way are a considerable advantage in treatment and an even greater advantage in chemoprophylaxis, which is undergoing an extensive field trial in Micronesia (Sloan *et al.*).

Sulfone resistance does evolve in a small percentage of cases. It is usually first suspected when the parameters of clinical improvement and decline of the BI or MI, or both, show no further improvement. It can be proven only by showing that organisms from the patient will multiply in mouse footpads despite protective administration of dapsone to the inoculated mice, a tedious and difficult procedure not practicable in most institutions.

RIFAMPICIN

In 1957, Lepetit in Milan, Italy, found an antibiotic in cultures of *Streptomyces mediterranei,* which he named rifamycin. From this has been developed rifampicin, known in the United States as rifampin, and marketed as Rifadin® (Dow) or Rimactane® (Ciba). It has been approved by the FDA for use against tuberculosis. It has been found clinically and bacteriologically effective against leprosy in Malaysia, and Shepard has found it far more rapidly effective against *M leprae* in the mouse than any other drug so far studied.

In a group of patients with leprosy at the USPHS Hospital in San Francisco, treated with 600 mg of rifampin daily, infectivity of their organisms for the mouse footpad disappeared completely by the seventh day of treatment, while with dapsone, more than 50 days are required.

Thus for the first time in the history of chemotherapy of leprosy, we have two effective drugs: a rapidly acting bactericidal one, rifampin, and a more slowly acting bacteriostatic one with known effectiveness over long periods, dapsone. A combination of these is being tried at the USPHS Hospital in San Francisco: 1500 mg of rifampin given orally once every three months, plus 50 mg dapsone daily. Shepard has suggested 1500 mg of rifampin and 225 mg of DADDS, each being given every three months. We feel that the combination of rifampin and dapsone or perhaps acetyl dapsone is most promising.

OTHER ANTILEPROTIC DRUGS

Thiambutosine, or Ciba 1906, a thiocarbamide derived from diphenylthiourea, is moderately effective against leprosy (Davison thinks it as effective as dapsone) in a dose of 2 gm a day for an adult. Drug resistance against it has been observed. It cannot yet be sold or dispensed in America.

Clofazimine (Lamprene or B663 Geigy), a riminophenazine derivative, developed by Vincent Barry of Dublin, is bacteriostatic against *M leprae* and also anti-inflammatory, in doses of 100 mg one to three times daily. It has an important and objectionable side effect: staining of the involved skin from brown to greyish-blue, most severely in light-exposed areas, often lasting for years after treatment is stopped. Its main use is in dapsone-resistant leprosy, and in patients having severe lepra reactions, particularly erythema nodosum leprosum. The dose should probably never be higher than 200 mg daily and for maintenance therapy, 100 mg twice a week.

Ethionamide, an isonicotinic acid derivative, has limited usefulness in dapsone resistance, in a dose of 250 mg three times a day. It is only bacteriostatic, and should not be used alone, but preferably with rifampin or clofazimine.

COMPLICATIONS AND REACTIONS

Dapsone in the doses used in leprosy rarely causes either methemoglobinemia or hemolysis, and though it may gradually induce anemia or leucopenia this is very unusual, and routine blood counts are not usually done. Lowering the dose of dapsone, or interrupting treatment for a few weeks, may be necessary if anemia should occur. The dose can almost always be gradually restored to the optimal level.

A true allergic drug eruption is rarely caused by dapsone, but if this does happen it may be impossible to continue the drug.

Albuminuria may also occur, but if there is no other evidence of renal insufficiency, dapsone need not be stopped.

Almost all leprosy workers mention psychosis as an occasional complication of sulfone therapy, but this must be extremely rare. We have not seen it.

LEPROSY REACTIONS

Lepra reactions (in lepromatous leprosy) and tuberculoid reactions may occur during sulfone therapy, but occur in untreated patients too, and are so common that we agree with Guinto and Binford that they should be considered as part of the disease rather than a complication of treatment.

Thalidomide, introduced by Sheskin and Sagher in Israel for the treatment of lepra reactions, is even more effective than corticosteroids in the alleviation of ENL. Its use in the United States is severely restricted by the FDA to a few institutions, because of its teratogenic potentiality. In a dose of 100 mg one to three times a day, it is effective in suppressing attacks, and 100 mg once a day is usually sufficient to prevent recurrences. In women who might possibly be pregnant and cannot safely be given the drug, either oral prednisolone, 40 to 60 mg a day, gradually tapered off, or intramuscular triamcinolone acetonide (Kenalog IM), 40 to 80 mg, repeated after a few days if necessary, may be used. Adding clofazimine (B663 Geigy) may help too, because of this drug's anti-inflammatory effect. As a rule, however, ENL should not be considered an indication for stopping sulfone therapy or even reducing the dose.

MAINTENANCE THERAPY

Most leprosy workers believe that lepromatous patients need maintenance therapy for life, and although there is no general agreement regarding the optimal dose, we believe 50 mg of dapsone twice a week is sufficient for this purpose.

A recovered tuberculoid patient can probably be adequately protected by 25 mg twice a week, and we may ultimately be able to say that he can safely discontinue this after two, five, or ten years. At present no one can confidently say how long it should be continued.

PROPHYLAXIS

THE original method of prophylaxis against leprosy—isolation of all lepromatous cases, at least in endemic areas—is now virtually obsolete as a result of our new awareness that contagiousness declines rapidly during the first few weeks of sulfone therapy.

The second method, BCG inoculation, was proposed by Fernandez in 1939; he found that conversion from negative to positive lepromin reactivity occurred more regularly after BCG inoculation—and lasted longer—than the tuberculin conversion for which it was originally proposed. This method of prophylaxis has had a surprisingly up-and-down course, being apparently very successful in Brazil and Argentina, then rather unsuccessful in field trials by Bechelli in Burma, and at this writing it still occupies no well established place in our armamentarium. It should probably be used only with other measures, in parallel with chemoprophylaxis, where maximum protection is desired for a susceptible contact or contacts: for example, if accidental inoculation with infective material has occurred. In such a situation 1500 mg of rifampin should also be given and should be repeated every three months for two years along with the usual dapsone prophylaxis.

The third method, chemoprophylaxis, is the most important one. Dharmendra demonstrated in India, in 1969, the effectiveness of prophylactic administration of dapsone in family contacts up to the age of 14 years. He gave dapsone twice weekly in slowly increasing doses to 569 contacts and a placebo to another 269, with a 12% incidence of leprosy in the latter against only 5% in the dapsone-treated group. Only one case occurred after the first year of prophylactic treatment.

We advocate prophylactic treatment for all close contacts of patients with lepromatous leprosy. "Close contacts" means family members or household contacts who show no evidence of leprosy. It is probably especially important for children. A dose of 50 mg twice a week for an adult, and for children correspondingly less according to age: twice weekly doses of 2 mg for an infant, 10 mg for a three-year-old, 15 mg for a six-year-old, 25 mg for a ten-year-old and so on. We suggest that this be continued for two years, at which time it can be stopped if the contact shows no evidence of having been infected, though periodic ex-amination of the contacts should be continued annually for ten years.

The effectiveness of Hanselar®—diacetyl dapsone—in doses of 225 mg every eleven weeks, in chemoprophylaxis of leprosy, has been established for small isolated population groups by Sloan *et al.* and it seems likely that the future will see much wider use of this convenient drug for this purpose and probably also for maintenance therapy of arrested cases of leprosy.

REHABILITATION

Rehabilitation, in the strict sense of restoration of damaged hands and feet to a more functional state, is beyond the scope of this book. The services of physical therapists, and orthopedic and plastic surgeons, are necessary. The following statement stressing the principles of prevention of deformity is taken from recommendations made by Dr. Oliver W. Hasselblad, President of American Leprosy Missions, in a report regarding the management of leprosy in Vietnam, which, however, apply all over the world.

> Prevention of deformity must begin at the time of diagnosis and become as vital a part of therapy as the specific medication. This can only be accomplished by persistent teaching and demonstrating to the patient that the smallest wound or injury to an area of anesthesia must be taken seriously; he must understand that the injury is self-inflicted. To prevent more serious developments in hands and feet that may be both anesthetic as well as having varying degrees of paralysis, the patient must be taught to avoid misuse of the affected parts. Simple measures including examination of anesthetic areas for signs of early injury, soaking and oiling dry skin of hands and feet, simple exercises to maintain mobility of affected

limbs and prevention of fixed deformity must all become a part of the daily life of the patient. All of this takes time, patience, skill, and persistent teaching.

Hasselblad calls plantar ulcers one of the most critical complications and states "A very simple type of foot-wear using the proper shore of microcellular rubber can prevent a high percentage of the plantar ulcers that would otherwise occur in anesthetic feet."

Advice for special problems can be obtained from Dr. Paul Brand, at the U. S. Public Health Service Hospital, Carville, La. 70721, and from Dr. Oliver W. Hasselblad, American Leprosy Missions, 297 Park Avenue South, New York, N.Y. 10010, who have developed rehabilitation services to a very high level. The authors can be queried on any problems at Straub Clinic, Honolulu, Hawaii 96813 (HLA) or USPHS Hospital, 15th Ave. & Lake St., San Francisco, Calif. 94118 (PF).

INDEX

89